Social Work
in Rural Australia

Social Work
in Rural Australia

Enabling practice

Edited by Jane Maidment and Uschi Bay

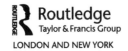

Routledge
Taylor & Francis Group

LONDON AND NEW YORK

First published 2012 by Allen & Unwin

Published 2020 by Routledge
2 Park Square, Milton Park, Abingdon, Oxon OX14 4RN
605 Third Avenue, New York, NY 10017

Routledge is an imprint of the Taylor & Francis Group, an informa business

Editorial arrangement copyright © Jane Maidment and Uschi Bay 2012
Copyright © individual chapters remain with authors

Cataloguing-in-Publication details are available
from the National Library of Australia
www.trove.nla.gov.au

Index by Puddingburn
Set in 11/13 pt Sabon by Midland Typesetters, Australia

ISBN-13: 9781742373706 (pbk)

CONTENTS

CONTRIBUTORS

Margaret Alston OAM is Professor of Social Work and Head of the Department of Social Work at Monash University in Melbourne, where she established the Gender, Leadership and Social Sustainability (GLASS) research unit. Her research interests are gender, social work, rural issues and climate change.

Uschi Bay is a Senior Lecturer in Monash University's Department of Social Work. Her research area is community sustainability, and so far her research has focused on desert and coastal communities in Australia. Uschi is an active member of the Gender, Leadership and Social Sustainability (GLASS) research unit at Monash University.

Liz Beddoe is an Associate Professor of Social Work in the School of Counselling, Human Services and Social Work at the University of Auckland. Liz has long-standing interests in critical perspectives on social work education, professional supervision in health and social care, the sociology of professions, the professionalisation project of social work, interprofessional learning and practitioner research.

Wendy Bowles is an Associate Professor at Charles Sturt University, Wagga Wagga. She has been a social worker, mostly in the disability field, since 1980. Since moving to a rural and academic life, her teaching and research interests have covered the broad terrain of social work theory, practice and ethics, with a focus on rural and regional practice.

Linda Briskman is Professor of Human Rights Education at Curtin University in Perth. Her main fields of advocacy and research are Indigenous rights and asylum-seeker rights. Publications include *Social Work with Indigenous Communities* (Federation Press, 2007) and *Human Rights Overboard: Seeking asylum in Australia* (Scribe, 2008, with Susie Latham and Chris Goddard), which won the 2008 Australian Human Rights Commission award for literature.

Mollie Burley is the Interprofessional Collaboration Team Leader at Monash University's Department of Rural and Indigenous Health, Moe, Victoria. She also works as a consultant in La Trobe Community Health Service, focusing on increasing and enhancing student placements, and facilitating education and research for staff—all underpinned by an interprofessional collaborative practice model.

Lesley Chenoweth is Professor of Social Work and Head of Logan Campus at Griffith University, Brisbane. From her early years as a social worker in rural Queensland, her research has focused on rural service delivery and rural practice.

Suzanne Hodgkin is a Senior Lecturer in Social Work and Social Policy in the La Trobe Rural Health School, La Trobe University, Bendigo, Victoria. Her practice experience is in family and children's services. She researches in the areas of gender, social capital, ageing and intergenerational care.

Yvonne Jenkins is a founding member of a rural housing cooperative (1996) and long-time board member of the Association of Resource Co-operative Housing (ARCH), the peak New South Wales statewide body advocating for rental housing cooperatives. Yvonne graduated with a Graduate Certificate in Housing Management and Policy at the Swinburne Institute for Social Research in 2002.

David McCallum is Associate Professor and coordinator of Sociology at Victoria University in Melbourne. His recent research interests have included historical studies of childhood behaviour disorders and the history of Aboriginal child removal in Victoria. He is a member of the Sociological Association of Australia and the Research Group in Sociology of Law of the International Sociological Association.

Jane Maidment is a Senior Lecturer in Social Work at Christchurch Polytechnic Institute of Technology in New Zealand. She previously spent ten years working in Australia. Jane has research and writing interests in field education, practice skills, ageing, and using craft as a vehicle for social connectedness.

Robyn Mason is a Senior Lecturer and social worker with practice experience in rural Australia. Her doctoral research was based on a national study of rural women's support services. She is currently based at Monash University, and is National Director of the Australian Association of Social Workers (AASW).

Jeni Warburton is the John Richards Chair of Rural Aged Care Research at La Trobe University in Wodonga, Victoria. Jeni has over 20 years' experience in research into social policy, healthy productive ageing, volunteering and the community.

Sarah Wendt is a Senior Lecturer in the School of Psychology, Social Work and Social Policy and a member of the Research Centre for Gender Studies at the University of South Australia. Her research interests are violence against women, child sexual assault, elder abuse and rurality.

PART I

Introduction

1

UNDERSTANDING RURALITY: A CONCEPTUAL FRAMEWORK

Jane Maidment

CHAPTER OBJECTIVES

- To outline the aims and scope of this publication.
- To explore the diverse and complex nature of rurality.
- To examine mythology and discourse related to rural Australia.
- To canvass rural practice and policy implications.

INTRODUCTION

Images of parched land and water towers and of rugged men wearing Akubra hats adorn websites dedicated to portraying rural Australia. Phrases such as the 'sunburnt country', made famous in Dorothea MacKellar's poem 'My Country', and the 'tyranny of distance', captured in Geoffrey Blainey's thesis on how distance has shaped Australian history, are some of the most abiding images of the Australian landscape presented in the written literature. Yet a closer examination of rural Australia provides evidence of a population, setting and practice context much more diverse and complex than these iconic representations suggest. In this book, we canvass the varied nature of Australian rural living and working, with particular reference to how this context shapes and informs social work practice.

The first section of this chapter briefly explains how this publication might be used by practitioners, educators and students interested in rural Australia and social work practice. This section provides an outline of the aims and scope of the publication and an overview of the organising framework used to inform the structure and pedagogy of the book. It concludes with a brief explanation of nomenclature used in the text.

The second and more substantive section of the chapter addresses the definitional complexity associated with understanding notions of regional, rural and remote Australia. It examines features of rural Australian demography, noting the nature of diversity encountered in these regions; provides an overview of the abiding mythology and discourse related to these parts of the country; illustrates the role that technology and innovation have played in changing the lived experiences and work practices of those residing in rural and remote communities; and concludes with an overview of how the contextual factors discussed above influence social work practice and policy development in rural Australia.

AIMS, PURPOSE AND LANGUAGE

The principal aim of this book is to provide a counter-story to the 'normalised' view of social work education as an urban phenomenon, taught predominantly from city campuses where urban-centric views of practice, policy and ethics prevail. In this text we are seeking to explore how social work practice in rural and remote Australia differs from that found in urban and regional spaces, with a view to equipping students to be more informed about practice issues and policy challenges encountered in rural work.

Previous literature on rural social work has identified that practitioners in this context need to find ways to sustain themselves professionally, manage high visibility and accessibility in a small community, and develop ways to establish and maintain a work–life balance (Lonne & Cheers, 2001; Green, 2003). Earlier studies report that social work practitioners experience poor levels of adjustment when they have not previously lived or worked in a rural area (Zapf, 1993; Lonne, 2003). Together, these findings strengthen the case for increased curriculum content on rural practice, policy and research within social work education, to better prepare graduates for working in this context.

A second aim of this book is to demonstrate the diversity of rural livelihood options and lifestyles found in rural and remote regions of Australia, and examine the subsequent implications for social work practice. Rural living and work options in this country have principally been shaped by features of geography, including topography, climate, and the presence of minerals and other natural resources. Each of these contexts provides different challenges to those living and working close by, and influences the ways in which practice and policy needs are expressed and the subsequent response. As such, the purpose of Part II of this book is to present the key concepts of understanding the notion of rurality, examining the construct of livelihood and engaging with interprofessional education.

Each of the chapters in Part III introduces readers to a specific type of livelihood context and field of practice. Within these chapters, particular attention is paid to making overt connections between potential practice issues encountered in the field, with macro socio-political concerns emanating from the policy and locational context (mining town, agricultural community, desert settlement). The last chapter, in Part IV, is designed to provide an agenda for future practice and policy development in rural Australian social work. This chapter is written to signal areas for potential growth, innovation, challenge and change for social work as a discipline. With this in mind, Chapter 15 is intended to create a platform for debate and engagement in Australian rural practice policy and development.

RURAL AND REMOTE AUSTRALIA: A DEFINITIONAL CONUNDRUM?

The question of defining rurality is complex. For functional purposes, the Australian Standard Geographical Classification (ASGC) system has formed the basis for Australian Bureau of Statistics (ABS) statistical data collection since 1984. The demarcations of measurement for this system are divided into spatial units, with one being dedicated to a calculation of remoteness in order to help inform Australian policy development (ABS, 2007a: 2). This system has recently been reviewed with an updated version renamed the Australian Statistical Geography Standard (ASGS), implemented from July 2011 (RDAA, 2010). The ASGC provides a simple measure of geography and is not designed to provide socio-economic data, information about access to vital services or analysis of the types of populations typically living in a given area (RDAA, 2010). Thus using a classification system like the ASGC, which focuses on aspects of physical geography to define rurality, is flawed in terms of helping to gain an understanding of the lived experiences of those residing outside urban centres.

Richard Pugh and Brian Cheers (2010) offer alternative ways to conceptualise rurality. Within the confines of social work practice and policy, these authors distinguish between examining rurality first in terms of setting and context, and second in relation to the type of social work practice and policy initiatives undertaken in the field. In this vein, key features of what rural and remote practice may entail are identified (2010: viii). This delineation is helpful since the notion of context and setting lends itself to inclusion of diverse livelihoods and geographies, while practice and policy modalities speak to the range of knowledge, skills and values that will be necessary for engaging with rural people and their issues. Neither interpretation assumes a universal standard of what 'rural' looks like, instead providing space for diverse intervention possibilities that inevitably will be shaped by changing social, economic and political circumstances and influences.

The way in which rurality is understood is also entirely dependent upon the lived experience of an individual or group engaged within this context at a particular point in time. Andrew Gorman-Murray (2009) makes this point particularly well in his examination of how the meaning of 'Chill Out', Australia's largest rural gay, lesbian, bisexual, transgender and queer (GLBTQ) festival, is interpreted quite differently by individuals who attend the festival from rural and urban areas:

> While the rurality of the festival is crucial for all, its meanings and experience shift across groups: urbanites invoke the idyllic country setting as a place to 'chill out', while rural residents stress the politicised catalysing effect of having a GLBTQ festival in a rural place. (2009: 71)

In this vein, it is clear that the meaning and analysis of what rural is and how it is understood can shift, change and differ in subtle ways, depending upon the positioning of whoever is offering the interpretation.

RURAL DEMOGRAPHY

From a demographic perspective, Australia's population reached an estimated 21.96 million in June 2009, with significant growth in New South Wales, Queensland and Victoria. This population increase has occurred predominantly in the inner city, outer suburbs and along the coastline, while population decline is evident in inland, rural and mining regions (ABS, 2010b). Even so, 14 per cent of the Australian population live in settlements of fewer than 1000 people

(ABS, 2002), with 22 per cent of the Aboriginal population living in outer regional areas, 10 per cent in remote areas and 16 per cent in very remote areas (HREOC, 2008).

The population decline in inland areas, brought about as a result of drought, bushfires and changes in mining activity, is of particular note in these figures. A significant feature of the internal migration has been the movement of younger people to the coast and city regions to gain education and work opportunities. This pattern has resulted in the growth of an aged cohort among those choosing to remain in rural and remote regions. The uneven distribution of population by age has resulted in labour shortages for farm work, with the ageing farming population living longer and continuing to farm until later in life (Barr, 2010). Meanwhile, this same aged cohort is providing care to grandchildren in order to enable other family members to work off drought-affected farmlands (Alston & Kent, 2004). The multiple demands experienced by this population, in conjunction with declining farm incomes and the need to diversify income sources (Pugh & Cheers, 2010: 15), have led to significant changes in land-management practices, and influenced associated family decision-making and succession planning. This cluster of dynamics impacts greatly upon family livelihood and well-being for those living in rural communities, and has important implications for the ways in which social work services are focused and delivered.

Another significant demographic trend includes the marked decrease in the number of young women participating in farming activity, who instead are moving to urban areas to pursue career and educational goals. The migration of women from rural areas has led to the masculinisation of the agricultural sector, and a gender imbalance within rural populations (Barr, 2010). Small rural communities throughout Australia have endeavoured to address this social issue by encouraging single women to visit their regions and meet locals through the provision of farm stays and weekend retreats, and hosting social functions such as dances for single people. At the same time, the popular Australian television program *The Farmer Wants a Wife* has publicised the phenomenon of isolated farmers needing and looking for a life partner. Numerous online websites focused on rural dating opportunities have sprung up in response to the problem of isolation and gender imbalance in the bush. While these activities often result in wry grins from viewers and readers, there is a serious side to attracting women to live outside urban areas, with the sustainability of rural and remote communities throughout Australia being contingent upon population regeneration.

From the late 1990s, new migrants to Australia have also actively been directed by the Department of Immigration to settle in rural areas through the development of new visa pathways. The purpose of this policy initiative has been to help repopulate these regions and provide essential labour and skills (Collins, 2010; Sivamalai & Nsubuga-Kyobe, 2009). Labour shortages of doctors and nurses, welders, mechanics and unskilled people to do fruit picking and other manual work are evident in rural communities. People from diverse cultural backgrounds have a long history of being resident in rural and regional Australia, dating back to the arrival of the Chinese during the gold rush years in the second half of the nineteenth century. Stereotypical assumptions might be made about the redneck nature of rural communities and the potential for migrant populations to experience discrimination (Pugh & Cheers, 2010); however, findings from research into the experience of migrant populations moving into rural areas suggest that recent newcomers have been made to feel welcome, with new Australians reporting high satisfaction levels in relation to lifestyle, climate, environmental physical surrounds, schooling options and work opportunities. Access to public transport and entertainment options in rural Australia was rated by overseas migrants as being less satisfactory (Collins, 2010). A more detailed analysis of the experience of migrants to rural Australia, and the implications for social work policy and practice, can be found in Linda Briskman's discussion on this topic in Chapter 10.

DIVERSITY

While rural and remote Australia is home to diverse populations, the landmass itself is also characterised by diverse topography, geography, climate and the livelihood options these features support. Australia includes large tracts of desert, mainly located in Western Australia, the Northern Territory and South Australia, punctuated by very small towns or settlement populations; rural communities dominated by the presence of the mining industry, such as Mount Isa in Queensland, Kalgoorlie in Western Australia and Coober Pedy in South Australia; farming and cropping districts such as the large Western Australian wheatbelt and the sugar cane plantations in northern New South Wales and Queensland; communities focused on fishing and aquaculture, with this business ranked the fifth most valuable Australian rural industry after wool, beef, wheat and dairy (Department of Agriculture, Fisheries and Forestry, 2010); and small boutique towns such as Bright (Victoria), Mapleton (Queensland) and Richmond (Tasmania), located within striking distance of a city and thus predominantly catering for the 'tree-changer' population, those wishing to escape the pressures of city living (Salt, 2009) while remaining within commuter distance of urban workplaces.

The last four decades have witnessed unprecedented change within rural communities. These changes have been prompted by economic and technological shifts with declining terms of trade for Australian agricultural products impacting upon the sustainability of small farm holdings. Pressure to increase farm productivity has resulted in a steady buy-up of land between farming neighbours, resulting in the disappearance of many small family farms. This phenomenon has been observed keenly by social researcher Neil Barr:

> Neighbour watches neighbour, assessing which farm will come onto the market and when this might occur. Those businesses that do not increase their productivity and fall behind are likely candidates. Those businesses that lack a successor are likewise potential targets. And so, the business and family life of neighbours is of business interest to the ambitious farming family. Poor farm management, farming or personal misfortune, inability to partner, infertility or descendents with aspirations other than farming—all are potential long term opportunities for neighbours. (Barr, 2010: 10)

The need to increase farm productivity is further acknowledged and encouraged by national farm awards dedicated to diversification, where a recent winner from New South Wales farmed an operation that included a large beef enterprise, growing timber for firewood and high-quality cabinet-making, a truffle industry, native grass-seed production, bed-and-breakfast accommodation and farm visits (Gocher, 2010).

Small rural towns that were in a state of economic decline during the 1960s have been regenerated through the migration of 'alternative lifestylers' from the city seeking low-cost housing and closer proximity to features of the natural environment (Sherwood, 2000). The challenge to established lifestyles and values brought about by the integration of new and diverse populations with long-term residents has inevitably been experienced by some as an initial confrontation of difference. There are, however, numerous examples where disquiet and difference have been transformed into mutual respect, positive gains and 'high-synergy' transactions, leading to the economic and social revitalisation of rural towns (Sherwood, 2000: 39; Frost, 2006).

A drive towards commercial and trade diversification in rural Australia has led to a growing range of enterprises using small towns as a focal point. Examples of these include the emergence of tourist shopping villages located in areas of historical interest, such as Yackandandah in the old Victorian goldfields and Evansdale in Tasmania, with its associated convict history. In this regard, the economic activity of shopping has become integral to the maintenance and preservation of the cultural heritage tourism industry (Frost, 2006).

Rural communities have also taken to hosting a diverse range of festival activities to bring people to the region and showcase local produce, horticulture, services, music, arts and crafts. Festivals have proven to be 'lively cells of economic activity' in small local economies, contributing in a small way to job creation while providing impetus for strengthening social capital through high rates of participation in volunteer activity (Gibson, 2008). For some communities, ongoing festival activity helps to sustain the local economy, with one example being the small town of Wakool in New South Wales. This town, with its population of just 4800, hosted 22 festivals during 2006–07 (Gibson, 2008). For other communities, large one-off events such as the iconic race day in Birdsville, Queensland, supply an annual injection of capital into the local economy. During 2010, the cancellation of race day due to heavy rain was a very real financial blow for the Birdsville community.

A growing number of food and wine trails found in inland regions are evidence of additional rural business diversification. The success of such trails is dependent upon numbers of small businesses working cooperatively together to market the region and a range of diverse products. Development of tourism through the mechanism of a trail involves not only the selling of products at particular destinations but the marketing and upkeep of the scenic surrounds and points of historical interest on the trail (Mason et al., 2008). For this reason, some in the wine industry who see their business and vocation primarily as growers and producers of fine wine dislike being part of the trail enterprise, even though it is an economic necessity. These growers associate the trails with the business of tourism and not prestige viticulture (ACIL Tasman, 2002), with different attitudes towards tourism creating some dissonance.

The Australian mining industry has spawned yet another unique type of rural settlement. Changes in industrial relations and employment conditions have produced an increased trend towards block shiftwork patterns in the mining industry, supporting a mobile fly-in/fly-out (FIFO) labour force, largely housed in work camps, company-owned single-person quarters, motel/hotel accommodation and caravan parks (Petkova et al., 2009). The transient nature of these town populations, the twelve-hour work rosters, physical tiredness and associated poor-quality family time impact upon the capacity of mine workers and their families to form meaningful social connections with each other and within the community (Lovell & Critchley, 2010). Having a mobile population tends to compromise the development of an infrastructure of public amenities such as child care, education and medical services in these towns. Those organisations reliant on volunteer input, such as the State Emergency Services (SES), community clubs and charity enterprises, struggle to survive in these communities, where the mobile workforce is not particularly invested in the ongoing development and future of the town (Pugh & Cheers, 2010).

These examples provide just a narrow illustration of the diverse range of lifestyle influences evident in different parts of rural Australia. The necessary forms of interdependence now needed among rural people to support production from these varied enterprises have resulted in shifts and changes within local networks, necessitating a renegotiation of alliances and relationships between diverse stakeholders (Boxelaar et al., 2007).

MYTHOLOGY AND DISCOURSE

Popular images of rural and remote Australia struggle to portray the diversity of both the lived experiences and physical geography of this vast continent. The character of rural and remote living differs considerably depending upon the landscape and nature of the context in question, with the notion of rurality predominantly serving as a cultural construct and spatial imaginary fulfilling a range of purposes in contemporary society (Gorman-Murray, 2009).

Even so, popular media, literary and artistic images generally speak to the tale of 'the outback and the bush', where the archetypes of rural and remote Australian identity are portrayed as tough, unyielding characters—usually men—struggling against the odds and the forces of nature (Simmons, 2003). This singular, blunt generalisation of rural Australia as home of the masculine battler has reinforced the denial of landscape and occupational complexities outside the major Australian cities, where local identities are shaped by their own geographies and supporting primary livelihoods (Bell, 1973). As noted above, in this book we endeavour to address the diversity of livelihood and lifestyle that can be found in rural Australia, with analysis to examine how such differences impact upon social work practice.

The normative portrayal of Australians' rugged stoicism has emerged out of an historical context, one strongly influenced by the struggles experienced by colonial settler and early penal populations in their encounters with the harsh physical environment (McHugh, 2004). However, this depiction is not inclusive of the Aboriginal experience, which has been mostly invisible in discourses about rural or urban Australian living. The Indigenous experience has been shaped largely through the European colonisation of Australia, subsequent dispossession of land, systematic cultural destruction and removal of Aboriginal and Torres Strait Islander children from their families (Briskman, 2007, cited in Beddoe & Maidment, 2009: 19), rendering this population disempowered, unseen and silenced in the portrayal of popular national character until very recent times.

Women, too, have historically been rendered invisible in portrayals of the Australian rural landscape. Most recently the archetype of rural Australia being the heart of Australia's 'blokeland' has been questioned in some mining communities, where efforts have been made to design more 'family-friendly' townships (Lovell & Critchley, 2010: 128), and women residents are expressing a sense of agency and control, contrary to earlier research that highlighted considerable levels and sources of female oppression (Gibson, 1994; Williams, 1981).

Notions of national identity have been fuelled by contemporary references in both the media and parliament to ideas or actions being 'un-Australian'. This potent colloquialism has appeared most recently in all manner of civic debate, ranging from the possible strike action of the national soccer team (Passant, 2009) to the potential loss of general practitioner services in a small rural community (Rule & Silvester, 2010). The idea that particular behaviours may be judged to be 'un-Australian' suggests that in the minds of some there exists a set of normative Australian values that together shape a 'preferred' national identity. These values include demonstrating behaviour perceived as being fair, self-sufficient and egalitarian, as well as coping in an understated way. This selection of core beliefs has been central to forging a strong national identity, reinforcing associations with resilience within the 'bush' mythology and the notion of 'mateship' (Butera, 2008). Traditionally, 'mateship' has been the preserve of men, inferring a sense of class solidarity, with women's participation being that of an outside observer only. These depictions of identity have served to strongly influence Australian literature and film, discourse and language (Bell, 1973; Webster, 2008), and speak to iconic representations of rugged rural living. Parallel to this tableau of rugged Australian rural and remote struggle and challenge has existed an equally powerful metaphor of progress and change, witnessed in a history of successive milestone feats of engineering and technological development.

TECHNOLOGY

The continent's vast landmass, together with the diverse and extreme weather conditions encountered in Australia, have provided the impetus for a 'history of revolutions' (Schumpeter, 1942, cited in Barr, 2010), early innovation and adaptation in technologies for communication, farming, education and health practice. Historically, the development of refrigerated transport in the later part of the nineteenth century together with mid-twentieth-century advances in chemical engineering has resulted in expanded exporting markets and a jump in agricultural production for the rural sector (Barr, 2010).

Of particular significance for contemporary Australian rural and remote communities are emerging developments associated with biotechnology for creating new agricultural products, energy sources and specialised lubricants; nanotechnology creating new fibres and membranes to prolong the shelf life of fresh produce; and information technology and radio frequency technology for tightening food supply chains (Barr, 2010: 20).

The development of a national strategy for tackling effective information and communication technology (ICT) rollout has been the source of much political debate in recent years. Lobby groups such as the National Farmers' Federation (NFF) have advocated hard for better technical infrastructure in rural and remote regions, including increased network coverage and internet reliability to support farming endeavours, rural family health, education and information needs (Corish, 2005).

The ability to access reliable ICT to conduct farming business, along with the adoption of biotechnology and precision farming technology, has led to increased farming productivity while reducing inputs of capital and labour (Nossal, 2009).

In particular, access to robust telecommunications technology has enabled farmers to:

- monitor international market trends
- communicate and interact with participants throughout the agriculture supply chain—that is, from paddock to the consumer and beyond
- use futures and option contracts to hedge against international markets and exchange rate fluctuations
- access weather forecasts, utilise seasonal climatic tools and plan farm strategies accordingly
- implement precision farming techniques to improve efficiency and deliver improved natural resource management outcomes, and
- use satellite imagery for developing whole farm plans (Corish, 2005: 3–4).

During 2005, Australian farmers were able to produce twice as much output as their 1970 counterparts (Barr, 2010: 7). Meanwhile, the very low population density over large tracts of rural and remote Australia has created both the impetus for and practical difficulties in implementing high-speed internet connectivity (Jackson, 2009). The unveiling of the National Broadband Network (NBN) strategy in 2009 was heralded as 'the largest single national building infrastructure in Australian history' (Rudd et al., 2010). Attendant policy development and debate around this technology initiative have focused on whether the need for quality rural ICT is so necessary that the inevitable urban subsidisation of this scheme is warranted. This particular tension encapsulates an oft-visited and potentially divisive national debate between rural and urban Australians around who subsidises the livelihoods of whom. This debate has become increasingly more vociferous and one-sided as agriculture's share of the Australian market economy has fallen from 14 per cent to 4 per cent (Productivity Commission, 2005), together with declining population numbers in rural and remote communities leading to diminished power for the rural constituencies in federal parliament. The strength of urban votes has also impacted upon the uptake of other agriculture-related technologies, including the adoption of genetically modified (GM) cropping techniques (Tribe, 2005).

In relation to social work practice in health and social care, the use of ICT has changed the shape and potential of delivery, record-keeping and professional development opportunities (Maidment & Macfarlane, 2009), with promised greater simplicity, storage capacity, uniformity and efficiency for workers, making it easier to calculate workloads and throughput, and generate statistics on client populations and service effectiveness (2009: 98).

Over the last decade, increasingly diverse use has been made of tele-health practice possibilities, opening up the potential and capacity for client care to be conducted across large distances, using a range of technologies. The use of videoconferencing for client consultations and assessment, professional development and supervision has meant that once very isolated practitioners can now have access to up-to-date expertise, information, advice and support from colleagues around the country. In addition, professionals and consumers now have access to more than 100 000 e-health web resources aimed at providing increased efficiency in health care, improved quality of care and empowerment of patients/consumers (Harrison & Lee, 2006). More detailed information about how changing technologies have impacted upon ongoing practitioner professional development and teamwork possibilities is provided by Liz Beddoe and Mollie Burley in Chapter 3.

PRACTICE AND POLICY DEVELOPMENT IN A RURAL CONTEXT

Pugh and Cheers call for the 'rejection of a homogenised approach to policy and practice' (2010: 195), advocating for recognition of the distinctive nature of rural livelihoods with ensuing social issues being reflected in context-specific policy and practice responses. These responses are inherently difficult to achieve, however, when social work curricula, social policy planning and practice have tended to be universally urban-centric in their focus. From an urban perspective, issues for rural people are often understood from a discourse of 'locational disadvantage', with an emphasis on rural problems and deficits (Daley & Avant, 2004). In this text, we intend to both identify the integral role played by place, space and physical geography in shaping practice and policy, while ensuring that formative examples of rural social policy and practice innovation and diversity are also canvassed.

Throughout, authors will demonstrate that to practise effectively in rural and remote areas it is critical to gather a good understanding of the local history and culture. Location-specific history and culture shape local norms and expectations in relation to social service delivery. The influence of particular cultural antecedents, the impact of past severe weather events, personal and community tragedies such as mining or agricultural fatalities, and the unique demography of a region will together mould what is deemed important in terms of sustaining community well-being. For this reason, priorities for service delivery and help-seeking behaviours will be diverse among rural populations across Australia.

The previous research and literature does identify some key concerns for Australian rural communities. These include the challenges of successful recruitment and retention of a professional workforce (O'Toole et al., 2010); the impact of climate change on agricultural sustainability (Mullen et al., 2010); the ageing rural demography fuelled by an exodus of young people to urban regions (Alston, 2009a; Stehlik, 2009); the status of rural health, education, housing and transport infrastructure (Bailie & Wayte, 2006; Collits & Gastin, 1997).

Given the breadth of issues identified above, social work intervention in rural communities usually incorporates both a generalist approach in terms of working across several fields of practice (such as child protection and aged care) and generic methods (group work, case management and community development) (Pugh & Cheers, 2010). Practitioners who both live and work in a rural area need to straddle multiple personal and professional roles, sustain high levels of community visibility and learn to negotiate complex issues of confidentiality in their day-to-day living arrangements.

Significant levels of informal care are provided by family members, neighbours and others in rural communities, where notions of commitment, shared obligation and interdependence prevail. The role of the practitioner in this context is to respect and work alongside these informal networks, drawing upon teamwork principles in doing so. In this way, the nature of the relationship between practitioner and client, informal caregivers and other service providers is likely to look and feel a little different from that found in an urban setting. The tenor of personal local links, family ties and history will have a bearing on the working relationships a practitioner is able to form with others, as well as their credibility. The space between the domestic and professional spheres of the practitioner is likely to be more fluid in a rural context, requiring careful attention to negotiating implicit assumptions and expectations people in the community may have about a worker's role. Being particularly mindful of setting clear boundaries in a diplomatic way is integral to sustaining a satisfying personal life as a practitioner in a small community.

Paradoxically, these same challenges provide a rich source of professional enlivenment where rural social workers tend to have more freedom to respond to situations in diverse and innovative ways (Pugh & Cheers, 2010) than their urban counterparts. Shortcomings in professional infrastructure and resources encountered in rural locations are often addressed through developing creative community solutions using the skills and knowledge base of both formal and informal community networks. The notion of 'needs must' creates the impetus and culture for inventive and flexible problem-solving to occur in rural practice, where workers have the opportunity to extend the boundaries of their knowledge and skill through challenge and innovation.

Significant state government initiatives to support rural and regional development are occurring at a policy level across the country, and provide traction for social work intervention using a socio-political emphasis. Most recently, the Victorian state government released *Ready for Tomorrow* (Regional Development Victoria, 2010), a blueprint for regional and rural development. This proposal outlines future planning and strategies to strengthen infrastructure in regional and rural areas by increasing public and freight transport options, improving internet connectivity and capacity, supporting small-town sustainability initiatives, and boosting tertiary education opportunities. Specific projects mooted in this state plan include the continued development of rail services for northwest Victoria; generation of water savings within the state through completion of the next phase of the desalination plant and making repairs to the statewide leaky irrigation system; strengthening investment in landcare, Indigenous education initiatives, public dental services and aged care initiatives; developing early childhood services in seven towns; and supporting local life and events such as festivals and cultural and sporting enterprises (Regional Development Victoria, 2010). Such policy initiatives are fertile ground for social work influence, in terms of facilitating individual and community consultation and participation in their development and implementation phases.

This chapter concludes with the message that rural practice is both challenging and exciting, with the notion of rurality itself being contestable and dynamic. The scope for grappling with this concept is captured by Mormont, who notes that: 'Rurality is not a thing or a territorial unit, but derives from the social production of meaning' (Mormont, 1990, cited in Gorman-Murray, 2009: 73). We invite readers to canvass the multiple meanings and interpretations of Australian rurality within the context of diverse livelihoods. This examination will subsequently reveal how various influences shape rural social work practice and policy.

RECOMMENDED READING

Barr, N. (2010) *The House on the Hill*. Land and Water Australia in Association with Halstead Press, Canberra.

Pugh, R. & Cheers, B. (2010) *Rural Social Work: An international perspective*. Policy Press, Bristol.

PART II

Rurality, topography and populations

2

MAKING A LIVING IN DIVERSE RURAL AND REMOTE COMMUNITIES

Uschi Bay

Geography shapes life experiences, defines reality and influences vision.—Locke et al., 1998: 74

CHAPTER OBJECTIVES

- To articulate the relationship between critical ecological systems theory and an anti-oppressive and empowerment perspective with rural, regional and remote social work practice.
- To outline the use of a sustainable livelihoods five capitals framework as an analytic tool to focus engagement with remote and rural communities.
- To elaborate on current neo-liberal techniques for governing through community engagement and the implications for rural, regional and remote communities.

INTRODUCTION

Social work practice in rural and remote Australia takes place in dynamic settings where there are ongoing and dynamic struggles over resources and to attain ecologically, economically, politically and socially sustainable livelihoods. An historical, social, economic, political and ecological contextual understanding of specific geographical locations is called for in rural, regional and remote place-based social work. Indeed, rural and remote social work is credited with reminding social workers of the holistic and contextual nature of social work itself. To deal with this complexity, I propose combining a critical ecological systems theory with an anti-oppressive and empowerment perspective to frame the overall analysis of a specific rural, regional or remote setting. Then I propose using tools like the sustainable livelihoods 'five capitals' framework with the addition of cultural capital as a way to structure this task. The sustainable livelihoods framework does need to be applied flexibly and in collaboration with the 'community'. Furthermore, an analysis of current neo-liberal policies such as governing through community engagement adds to social workers' analysis of how rural, regional and remote settlements are perceived and problematised by various policies and through media reporting. These strategies are designed to enable social workers to practise effectively using a place-based approach.

Recently, Michael Kim Zapf (2009) has promoted a reconceptualisation of the systems theory 'person in environment' mantra with a metaphor that captures the interdependence of people and place. Zapf struggled to find an expression that did not continue the focus on individuals and environment as separate, and sought to equally value the environment in ecologically informed social work. He chose 'people as place' to capture the focus on the collective task of ecological thinking, emphasising people rather than the individual. He designated 'place' rather than environment, as it denotes a combination of location, meaning, geography and emotional significance 'that brings together the natural world and human history, activities, and aspirations' (2009: 189). Zapf sought to capture a relationship between people and place that did not reinforce a separation between them, or set up a binary where humans are primary and the environment secondary. Hence he chose 'as' to reflect the interrelations and interdependencies in this relationship. Zapf is promoting the idea that social workers develop a place-based model of social work which reprioritises ecological concerns.

In Australia, neo-liberal governmental policies over the last two decades have aimed to govern through constructing a notion of 'community' that is predefined and predetermined, and at times constructs residents' interests without place-based communities' engagement in self-determining their destinies. I aim to challenge this way of thinking about rural, regional and remote communities and to promote a 'whole of community' focus that recognises diversity within communities. I propose that incorporating sustainable livelihoods strategies flexibly into social work practice with communities offers a way to develop processes and projects that support the broadest notion of what Zapf (2009) means by 'living well in place'.

CRITICAL ECOLOGICAL SYSTEMS THEORY

Systems theory in social work focuses attention on the 'person in environment', and articulates levels of practice from individual, family, group and community to policy-making and advocacy. In recognising the interaction between these systems, rural and remote social workers further promote an analysis of the interrelations at each of these levels and their intersections. Newer ecological systems theory is also aiming to articulate people's embeddedness in their ecological or natural environments and the *'mutual* contribution and response of each to an unending transactional process' that is understood as totally interdependent (Rothery, 2008: 91, emphasis in original; Zapf, 2009).

The strength of systems theory is this openness to broad social, political, economic and ecological issues, and careful consideration of their interaction with people in specific geographic locations. Traditionally, systems theories have focused on adaptation in order to achieve a 'goodness of fit' between people and their environments. This did not necessarily address social inequality, social injustice and institutional racism and/or sexism. To include these concerns, critical ecological systems theory incorporates analysis of power relations, and also acknowledges the import of fairness of access to and distribution of resources.

Another essential ingredient in the reconceptualisation of systems theory is Zapf's (2009) call for prioritising the natural environment. Zapf argues that social work ought to retire the 'person-in-environment' founding metaphor and replace it with the more dynamic metaphor of 'people as place' to indicate the interdependence and inseparability of people and place. He argues for a place-based social work model that recognises geography and place attachment, one which accepts that identity is connected to place and seeks to incorporate a sense of responsibility and stewardship for a healthy physical environment. Zapf (2009: 183–5) argues for an ecological consciousness linked to traditional knowledges and a bringing together of sacred and daily life. He promotes a model of social work that focuses on people and place and on a new social work mission to learn to live well in place.

The sustainable livelihoods approach and the five capital assets analysis and development of social, financial, physical, natural and human capital offer a framework for thinking about what assets are available in particular settlements and encourages an exploration of the implications for people's ongoing sustainable livelihoods. Sustainability in Zapf's (2009: 185) terms indicates place-based concepts like ecological literacy, attentive living in place, nature-centredness and local life opportunities. Adding a critical lens focuses further attention on the equitable distribution of the five capitals for various sub-groups within a rural, regional or remote setting as well as the notion of a sustainable planet. The idea of living well in place incorporates 'social justice with environmental justice, human rights and environmental rights, and human responsibilities with environmental responsibilities' (Zapf, 2009: 191).

SUSTAINABLE LIVELIHOODS APPROACH

One of the tools for understanding 'rural and remote Australian regions as dynamic socio-ecological systems' is the sustainable livelihoods approach (Davies et al., 2008: 55). A sustainable livelihoods approach is applicable to social work in rural and remote settings as it calls for 'an integrated analysis of complex, highly dynamic rural contexts' that takes into account 'histories of places and peoples and their wider interactions with colonialism, state-making and globalisation' (Scoones, 2009: 13–14). According to Jocelyn Davies and Sarah Holcombe (2009), the sustainable livelihoods approach within a neo-populist, participatory and empowerment approach aims to 'reduce poverty and disadvantage by engaging local knowledge and resources equitably, and by promoting institutional change' (2009: 364–5). Neo-populism as an approach explicitly stresses respect for local knowledge; and is people-centred and participatory, in that local people are to determine their own priorities (Davies & Holcombe, 2009: 364). This emphasis on participatory processes with the aim of enabling communities to have effective control of their own destinies resonates with social work principles in community development that promotes 'practices and processes to engage with communities in ways that empower communities to take *collective responsibility* for their own development' (Kenny, 2006: 10, emphasis in original).

A focus on 'livelihoods' as an approach to rural development internationally re-emerged with an influential paper by Robert Chambers and Gordon Conway in 1992, according to Ian Scoones (2009: 3).

Scoones characterises the livelihoods approach as 'integrative, locally-embedded, cross-sectoral and informed by a deep field engagement and a commitment to action' (2009: 3). Deep field engagement in this context means social workers, community workers and researchers actually living in rural and remote communities for some time in order to understand better how a specific community operates in its context. Examples of the sustainable livelihoods approach can be traced back over at least 50 years in rural development, especially in Asia and Africa. This livelihoods approach articulates a commitment to action linked to strategies for poverty alleviation, especially in developing countries and by international non-government organisations like Oxfam, and organisations like the United Kingdom Department for International Development (DFID), the United Nations Development Programme (UNDP) and CARE.

The sustainable livelihoods approach was developed in relation to the concerns and tensions arising out of environmental issues and economic development projects in developing countries by, importantly, broadening the notion of development beyond conventional economic considerations of finance, paid employment, market production and consumption. It is understood by the World Commission on Environment and Development (WCED, 1987) that livelihood security is pursued in many ways by people, not just through jobs; these include 'ownership of land, livestock or trees; rights to grazing, fishing, hunting or gathering' (WCED, 1987) as well as other activities like craft activities or other cultural or traditional practices. In many smaller settlements in rural or remote Australia, 'regular'—or, as some politicians call them, 'real'—full-time jobs are rare and residents use various combinations of the five capitals to make a living in such places. People often combine various part-time jobs, casual and/or seasonal work to sustain or maintain themselves, their families and communities. Supplementation of income also includes growing food, gathering bush food, fishing, using natural materials to build houses or to make objects for use and bartering, as well as finding ways not to spend money on water and energy costs. Attracting tourists and tourist dollars through music festivals, sporting events, arts and craft are at times also very effective strategies by rural towns to draw financial and cultural capital. A broader definition of livelihood strategies is relevant for understanding rural and remote communities' livelihood practices.

The formal definition of sustainable livelihoods tends to focus more on the actual ongoing ability of people to continue making a living in a particular way in a specific place. A livelihood is said to be sustainable 'when it can cope with and recover from stresses and shocks and maintain or enhance its capabilities and assets both now and in the future, while not undermining the natural resource base' (Chambers & Conway, 1992: 7). This definition indicates the inter-relationship between natural resources and capabilities of people to adapt to changes. The 'stresses and shocks' may be sudden and temporary events or unexpectedly longer drawn-out events—some examples are the recent economic recession, floods, fires and ten-year drought, and incremental policy changes like the deregulation of dairy farming. However, with climate change impacting on the natural resource base over recent decades, in relation to reduced fish stock, soil salinity, water availability and variations in agricultural crop cycles, the notion of sustainable livelihoods now needs to take into account these effects on the natural resource base. These events challenge the kinds of livelihoods that can be sustainable in relation to changes in the 'natural resource base', whether in response to deplet-ing or degraded natural resources or due to wider human activity.

The sustainable livelihoods approach is not about measuring people and testing whether their livelihoods are sustainable; rather, as Davies and colleagues (2008) point out, 'it is a tool or a way of thinking designed to assist in identifying changes that can be made to institutions, to people's assets or their strategies in order to promote the resilience of local livelihood systems' (2008: 56). There is a central focus on the institutional aspects in the sustainability frame-work, and social workers using a critical ecological systems theory consider the structural aspects of livelihoods and recognise the impor-tance of facilitating empowering changes at this level. To understand rural, regional and remote Australian settlements, the sustainable livelihoods model focuses on the 'five capitals' asset model. This five capitals model has been used by the Desert Knowledge Cooperative Research Centre (DKCRC) in desert communities and the Centre for Appropriate Technology (CAT) in Alice Springs, as well as by social workers like Margaret Alston to systemically map the interre-lations of various influences on sustainability of livelihoods in rural Australia (Cocklin & Alston, 2003) and others.

The point of applying the sustainable livelihoods perspective to rural and remote Australian social work is to broaden the contextual frame to explicitly address several different dimensions of sustainability: 'the environmental, economic, social and institu-tional' (DFID, cited in Scoones, 2009: 10). It is all too easy, even though the sustainability livelihoods approach aims to 'bridge the gap' between macro and micro levels, to dump these macro concerns 'in a box labelled "contexts"' (Scoones, 2009: 11) in order to emphasise the local at the cost of dealing with the macro levels like global markets, economics, and ecological and political changes.

THE 'FIVE CAPITALS' ASSETS FRAMEWORK

A decade ago, the UK Department for International Development (DFID) developed the generic sustainable livelihoods framework (Scoones, 2009; Davies et al., 2008). The framework highlights the interaction between risks, the five capital assets, institutions, livelihood strategies and outcomes. This generic sustainable livelihoods framework was adapted by community developers, a range of researchers from different disciplinary backgrounds and specifically rural sociologists and social workers, as a conceptual tool to assist in comprehensively identifying the influences impacting on and interacting within rural, regional and remote settlements.

The five capitals assets framework refers to *social* capital (social networks and relationships of trust), *natural* capital (natural resource stocks, natural environment and features), *financial* capital (savings, income, credit), *physical* capital (transport, shelter, water, energy, communication) and *human* capital (skills, knowledge, leadership, labour). It is thought that people draw on the five capital assets to develop and maintain their livelihood strategies. The capital assets framework is considered better than income, consumption and employment as a way of understanding sustainable livelihood (Hocking, 2003). Rural, regional and remote residents draw on diverse assets, and develop or maintain their livelihood strategies, within the context of broader social, political, ecological and other factors (Davies et al., 2008: 56). However, as Scoones (2009: 8) highlights, the 'capitals' and 'assets' framework can focus the notion of sustainable livelihoods too narrowly on outcomes within economic terms. The sustainable livelihoods framework is much broader than just a focus on financial income, a job or paid employment.

The five capitals framework, including social, financial, physical, natural and human assets, offers a way of thinking about what livelihood strategies are available in a particular settlement. When social workers add a critical lens to this framework, it focuses attention on the equitable distribution of these capitals between various subgroups within a rural, regional or remote setting. Issues of human

27

rights, land rights and the historical effects of colonisation, as well as the ongoing dynamic power relations between residents, continue to influence livelihood strategies. Adding an ecological lens further focuses attention on the interaction between livelihoods and nature-based resources, and the relationship between the livelihood strategies and the stewardship of the natural environment for current and future generations. Decisions to alter practices to conserve natural resources can be made by local rural, regional and remote residents, or such decisions can be imposed by policy changes at the local, state or national level.

In short, a critical ecological systems theory approach can find in the sustainable livelihoods framework a systematic focus on the interaction between rural and remote settlements' assets, decision-making processes, practices and community residents' livelihood strategies. The framework also recognises the central role of institutional structures on rural, regional and remote settlements, and on the need for residents to understand and influence policy-makers and the processes that govern their lives (Scoones, 2009: 10). 'Institutions comprise rules, norms and shared strategies, whether developed locally and embedded in culture, or formulated at other levels in legislation and policy' (Ostrom, 2005, cited in Davies et al., 2008: 56–7). In order to be effective in engaging with rural and remote communities in dealing with institutions, policy-makers and policy changes, social workers need to call on their social and public policy analysis skills to articulate the overall policy directions in ways that empower communities to determine their destinies. Later in this chapter, a governmentality approach to community as a policy construct will be explored further.

HUMAN AND SOCIAL CAPITAL

Social workers tend to identify their roles and interventions mostly in relation to two of the five capitals: human capital and social capital. Social capital refers to three types of relationships: bonding, bridging and linking. *Bonding* is understood as close relationships between like-minded and similar people or equals who trust each other. *Bridging* social capital is between people who are not alike but who relate across difference while often residing in or near each other in the same settlement. *Linking* capital is understood as networks of people with access to power, influence and resources who usually do not reside in the local settlement. Linking capital is sometimes identified as crucial for people living in settlements that have a stigmatised identity (see Warr, 2005). Linking capital is said to enable people residing in these poorer rural, remote and regional areas to draw on resources external to their settlement, to assist them with livelihood strategies and to overcome poverty traps. Social workers using a critical ecological systems theory can use the different emphases of the three types of social capital to guide the focus of their engagement with rural and remote communities.

One of the subtleties of working with communities on their 'social capital' is that social workers need to be clear about the limits of the three aspects of social capital—bonding, bridging and linking relationships. For instance, rural or remote settlements can discursively be positioned by external governmental institutions as *lacking* in social capital and charged to develop their social capital with the expectation that making communities responsible for developing their social capital will resolve complex issues, including structural problems such as lack of transport, adequate housing and employment opportunities (Bay, 2009). 'Social capital' is a problematic notion, however, especially in the context of neo-liberal governance, because neo-liberalism tends to shift responsibility for rectifying structural inequalities to rural, regional and remote settlements. The emphasis in social capital on 'the intangible role relations of trust and mutuality within a place-based location play in sustaining or even reviving urban or rural communities' tends to distract attention from resource needs, like the need for public transport, or housing, or health care or child care (Weeks et al., 2003: 6). For instance, remote desert settlements have historically been massively under-resourced and the missions and reserves in desert Australia, established by churches and governments, are located far from easy access to transport routes, which limits trade opportunities. These are historical and structural obstacles to people seeking to make a living in these locations, which cannot adequately be addressed by increased bonds of trust between people alone (Briskman, 2007). There are power relations that influence access to land, water and other natural resources, and to physical resources like schools, public transport and child-care services. The availability of people with high levels of human capital is numerically lower in rural, regional and remote settlements. This can mean that small communities are reliant on a very small number of individuals with leadership skills, vision and drive. Bridging social capital, including knowledge of how to gain resources from corporations and governments at various levels, as well as gaining access to private financial assets within an area, may be limited to just a few key people. This reliance on a few key leaders can make rural and remote settlement viability vulnerable to the loss of these individuals, be they billionaire graziers or elders in homeland communities. Often, strengthening regional, rural and remote sustainable livelihoods relies on finding strategies that enable a collective sharing of such knowledge.

'The most widely accepted definition of social capital today is the ability to secure resources by virtue of membership in social networks or larger social structures . . . and the benefits of social capital are understood to accrue to the collective' rather than individuals (Shortall, 2004: 112). Social workers who focus their energies on developing 'social capital' with remote and rural communities need to do so in a way that does not reinforce structural inequalities or inadvertently blame members of a settlement for the long-term effects of historical events and previous government policies, or focus too exclusively on economic development. Yet all of this does not detract from the importance of ongoing trusting relationships that engender care between and for all members of a 'community', regardless of location.

Human capital is related on an individual level to educational attainment and capacity for leadership, as well as to the embodiment of a vision for a settlement. On a community level, human capital has been related to the notion of capacity-building. The World Bank, with its focus on strengthening governance, and the United Nations Development Programme's (UNDP) linking of capacity-building to sustainable development and environmental issues, focus on organisational sustainability and the building of institutional capacity to shock-proof local organisations against staff turnover or leadership loss. In desert settlements that are heavily reliant on specific elders and leaders for vision, cohesion and the capacity to negotiate with a wide range of government bodies, succession planning was identified as an institutional and settlement sustainability strategy. Similarly, such ideas also influence farming communities and the passing on of farms to family members.

The notion of involving local people more in the workings of their own communities and various community groups is considered a form of capacity-building. Local residents' understanding of governance processes is often encouraged through engagement in partnerships with governments around strengthening the ways in which formal or incorporated groups make decisions and act within the law. Critics of this approach indicate that much of the capacity-building undertaken by external organisations is restricted to training, and may be too instrumental in flavour to enhance community members' capacity to assess and value local community opportunities or the development of capacities to engage in livelihood strategies to enhance their sustainability, either institutionally or ecologically.

CULTURAL CAPITAL

There are proposals being made that culture should be an additional capital, and that the five capitals framework needs to become a six capitals framework by including culture (Throsby, 1999, cited in Davies et al., 2008: 60). The importance of cultural expression for the development of sustainable livelihoods strategies can readily be appreciated, as culture is also a resource on which people can draw. From a sustainable livelihoods perspective, 'traditional knowledge handed down through generations, such as natural resource management expertise' in, for instance, desert Australia, contributes another dimension to social and human capital that may add to social workers' understanding of and engagement with rural, regional and remote communities (Commonwealth Foundation, n.d.).

A further point is that culture relates to human rights, and the expression of a range of cultural voices supports diversity. There are complex issues that surround the lives of minority cultural groups in Australia around the notion of assimilation, self-determination and intergenerational relations. The ways in which social workers deal with culture, with young people from minority cultures seeking to adapt to both their family's background culture and Australian expressions of values, lifestyles and livelihoods, aim to translate into people having choices. One of the measures of oppression, according to Bob Mullaly (2002), is that little is known in the mainstream culture about the life and culture of minority or colonised groups in a society.

Aboriginal people in desert Australia residing on traditional lands regard their dynamic cultural practices as 'underpinning all aspects of livelihoods' (Davies et al., 2008: 59). 'Aboriginal people hope to retain ownership of the knowledge [in this instance, of bush foods] that has been passed to them from their parents and grandparents as a human and social capital asset and to share it on their own terms' (Davies et al., 2008: 60). Aboriginal people's aim of retaining local ownership of knowledge links cultural knowledge to human and social capitals, and further to human rights issues and claims. From an anti-oppressive and empowerment perspective, social workers need to be alert to the risk to cultural assets from mainstream economic development processes, including the possibility of patents being taken out on plant properties by industry, thus impacting on bush food knowledge held by Aboriginal peoples in desert Australia.

The lack of inclusion of cultural components in understanding livelihood strategies can hamper the usefulness of human and social capital development in rural, regional and remote settings, as 'it is a factor that influences all elements of livelihood sustainability' (Davies et al., 2008: 60).

INTEGRATED ANALYSIS OF RURAL AND REMOTE CONTEXTS

The anti-oppressive and empowerment perspective draws attention to relations of class, race, gender and ethnicity, and how structural arrangements reinforce people's differential access to resources and opportunities. A livelihoods approach focuses attention on how livelihoods are structured by these kinds of relations, including religion and cultural identity. Understanding these structures requires

> asking basic questions: who owns what, who does what, who gets what and what do they do with it? Social relations inevitably govern the distribution of property (including land), patterns of work and division of labour, the distribution of income and the dynamics of consumption and accumulation. (Scoones, 2009: 14)

The following case study illustrates this point well.

CASE STUDY
While taking part in a broader sustainable desert settlement study, social work researchers explored the possibility of an Aboriginal-owned tourist business in a remote area of Australia. The Australian tourism literature considers Aboriginal-owned tourist businesses to provide a potential livelihood strategy for Aboriginal people. One possibility discussed with Aboriginal leaders in a specific small town was making a sacred Aboriginal site available for tourists to visit. In asking the basic questions stated above—about who owns what, who does what,

who gets what and what they do with it—it became clear that the land on which the sacred site is located is currently the property of a white settler grazier who uses the land for grazing cattle. There is an unresolved native title claim being argued by the local Aboriginal people that may or may not specifically relate to this site. There are issues of land ownership and land rights that impact on the decisions by the local Aboriginal people about this site as a 'resource' for a tourism business. If access to the site was arranged, then in order to make the sacred site accessible to tourists, fencing would be required to protect the grazing cattle, as gates being left open could create problems for the current landowner. Whose responsibility would this fencing be and who would bear the costs?

Tourists who presently find out about the site and visit it are often not sensitive, and leave rubbish and alter the site by moving rocks or signing or tagging stones. This is disrespectful of the site and the culture of Aboriginal people, and increasing access to tourists would create maintenance work for whoever takes over management of the site. The possibility of charging an entry fee would require arrangements to collect the fee (if people would pay to access it), and how this would be resourced is an issue. The next issue is who would be involved in managing the site—there may be limitations as the sacred site is a designated male Aboriginal site, thus restricting Aboriginal women's access and presumably their ability to contribute to its management, at least at the actual site.

This case study illustrates the intersection of class, occupation, race, gender, cultural identity and the effects of power relations in a remote desert settlement in relation to exploring one possible new livelihood strategy. From a post-structural theoretical perspective, a crucial point to be made is that 'the forms of community regulations and access to resources are invariably wrapped up with questions of identity' (Peet & Watts, 2004: 25) and power relations.

When working with whole communities and taking a pluralistic approach, social workers need to reflect on the implications that access to resources is the result of ongoing dynamic power relations. 'Communities are internally differentiated in complex political, social and economic ways [and social workers] need to be sensitive to the internal political forms of resource use' (Peet & Watts, 2004: 25). Land rights, social justice and struggles for equality in particular places and spaces are informed by historical and structural policies, programs and institutions that have ongoing impacts on the kind of access to resources and support some groups have in devising livelihood strategies. Social workers will need to treat seriously 'the means by which control and access of resources or property rights are defined, negotiated and contested within the political arenas of the household, the workplace and the state', according to Richard Peet and Michael Watts (2004: 12).

The questions then are: what happens next in this case example? Who determines what happens next? How are different views and perspectives negotiated and who is involved in these negotiations? Social workers may have a role to play in sensitively making explicit the normative understandings of livelihoods to encourage deliberation of the political choices being made in relation to livelihood strategies. A key question from an anti-oppressive and empowerment framework relates to whether these arrangements are reinforcing current power relations. Also, what values might influence the next steps in these processes? Can a process of inclusive deliberating about various livelihood options be developed across various sub-groups in small settlements? In working out what to do, the complexity of sorting out the effects of power relations on how marginal groups perceive the determining or limiting factors that impact on their possible livelihood strategies may need some ongoing attention. Mullaly (2002) argues that marginal groups internalise oppression and that this can limit people's aspirations. The effects of power relations in a colonial setting like Australia, particularly in relation to Aboriginal people, mean that social workers need to be aware, when aiming to build linking social capital between the state and a community or settlement, that 'it is influence and prestige, coupled with authority and money which fundamentally frame the forms of governance and hence who participates and who benefits' (Peet & Watts, 2004: 26).

In some desert settlements with predominantly Aboriginal residents, the sustainable livelihoods framework was applied by Desert Knowledge Cooperative Research Centre researchers in a very flexible and participatory way. This approach meant that residents were engaged in collecting the data to produce an analysis of their livelihood strategies and thus promoted an intercultural exchange of knowledge-sharing. One of the outcomes of this work was learning how the relationship between social capital, human capital and cultural capital operated in relation to paid work very differently when Aboriginal people accessed further training and education. For instance:

> Aboriginal people reported that they began to work in a particular job, or to undertake particular activities in care of land and people, because they were nominated or 'picked' by someone else as the person who should do that job or role. (Davies et al., 2008: 58)

Once in this job or role, they undertook further training and education for the position or role. This is the reverse of the situation in other cultures, where skills and training are pursued by people prior to taking up a position or role, and individuals are encouraged to select their own occupations or vocations. The sustainable livelihoods approach, used flexibly, highlighted a relationship between social and human capital that is culturally informed in very specific ways in some remote desert settlements.

In this way, 'Livelihoods analysis . . . is not a neutral exercise, knowledge production is always conditioned by values, politics and institutional histories and commitments' (Scoones, 2009: 16). As with the notion of 'social capital', the implications of using a sustainable livelihoods framework to assess communities' vulnerabilities and strengths need to be explored carefully for its effects on depoliticising poverty and the possible shifting of responsibility for inequalities to the very groups who are most targeted by oppressive forces. Critical ecological systems theory, in conjunction with the anti-oppressive and empowerment perspective, offers social workers tools for thinking about the relationship between identity, power relations, knowledge and livelihoods.

Often, rural and remote communities' issues are problematised by policy-makers and desert settlements, and their numerous deficits are frequently highlighted in the media (Nimmo & Zubrycki, 2008; Carney, 2008). Binary discourses about 'dying town syndrome' are contrasted with the almost magical rural revival of other small towns (Ingamells, 2007). The discourse about the inadequacies and 'messiness' or chaotic character of desert settlements is contrasted with the possibilities for greater safety and better health that are evident in some homelands settlements (see Chapter 11). The ways in which rural, regional and remote communities are characterised, discussed, analysed and governed, often 'at a distance' from decision-making centres, is part of the contextual framework used by social workers when engaging with communities in analysing and deconstructing these dualisms to explore 'the range of positions that lie within and beyond' these constructions (Healy, 2005: 205). Through this type of analysis, an opportunity-centric perspective rather than a problem-centric approach can be articulated with various sub-groups in remote, regional and rural communities (Boyd & Bright, 2007).

GOVERNANCE THROUGH COMMUNITY ENGAGEMENT

Australian public and social policy has been informed by neo-liberalism for the last two and a half decades, and the notion of community engagement has become part of the armoury of governing 'at a distance', meaning that governments understand their role as one of facilitating communities to do it for themselves. The notion of 'community' itself has become shorthand in this ideology for shifting responsibility to individuals or 'communities' for their self-sufficiency while supporting the withdrawal of various resources and government services. Self-sufficiency is often something on which rural and remote people pride themselves, yet governmental neo-liberal ideological imposition of self-sufficiency alters the meaning of the term. 'Self-sufficiency' has become harder to achieve, due to the withdrawal and recentralisation of government services and the outsourcing of service provision. When applying for funding through competitive tendering processes, service providers can rarely justify service delivery to smaller towns or homelands in desert Australia as these tenders do not allow for any so-called inefficiencies in allocation of time and resources. When smaller places are offered fewer local services, people struggle to meet their various needs and smaller settlements can come to be considered less viable by both residents and service providers.

Community engagement—especially through partnerships between community organisations and government departments—is considered an ideal mechanism for directing or governing at a distance. However, as a mode of governance it relies on communities or citizens being keen to participate in partnerships with government. It also assumes that communities are homogenous or unified and, having a single agreed agenda, it relies on skills and knowledge about how government operates and on communities to be well organised and able to call on sound leadership. These assumptions are idealistic and do not reflect the complexity of rural, regional and remote communities.

COMMUNITIES ARE INTERNALLY DIFFERENTIATED

First, it is important to understand that communities are not homogenous—indeed, 'communities are internally differentiated in complex political, social and economic ways' (Peet & Watts, 2004: 25). All communities, regardless of size, are socially stratified, and often this is geographically indicated in the way that poorer people or people of colour live in one part of town while the white wealthier elite or professional service groups reside in another part of town. People's social and economic status can at times be ascertained by their address or proximity to desirable local features like the golf course, the beach or the river, and away from less desirable features like the railway line, factories or highways. Settlements also comprise different identity groups, usually based on occupation, race, ethnicity, age and gender. There are interrelations between and within these sub-groups within a community. Social workers often need to tread very carefully in rural and remote communities, as some relationships between people—including leaders of different sub-groups—span many years and various agendas.

Several people in towns or small settlements occupy leadership roles in relation to negotiations within and externally to the settlement. As social workers, we need to be sensitive to the internal political relations between and within various sub-groups and the differential access each of these groups may have to various kinds of resources, including decision-making, as well as to the more traditional social services like education, health and income support. From a critical ecological systems theory perspective and an anti-oppressive and empowerment approach, this means paying close attention to which people or sub-groups are not engaged in or left out of negotiations, and how this might be altered over time. When social workers come into a community and only focus on dealing with the identified leaders, what can be missed is that 'local community action is often local class action instigated by the articulate and wealthy residents' (Blackstock, 2005: 43).

Another key point is that 'communities are rarely corporate or isolated, which means that the fields of power are typically non-local in some way' (Peet & Watts, 2004: 25). Rural and remote communities in Australia are often identified by non-residents as socially and geographically isolated, but this is not usually how local residents see their situation. For instance, two of the small desert settlements I worked with had regular international contact and interactions with visitors from Korea, Japan and the United States, to mention just a few countries. The town had staff from mining companies surveying the surrounds and the town hosted teams for sporting and charity events, attracting people from all around Australia. Various professionals from locations around Australia staffed the local government offices, schools, police stations and health services for varying periods of time while developing their careers. Itinerant workers were a regular feature in some occupations, and there were other kinds of visitors and tourists. Fly-in/fly-out health, recreation and social work services were also evident. The leaders of the various sub-groups residing in the town also travelled to regional, national and international sites to negotiate for various benefits for the settlement in relation to income, land and cultural rights, and the provision of services. The interaction with people in other places was also facilitated by telecommunications, such as the internet and email, and even in very remote areas radios and satellite dishes made communications possible. This means that an analysis of power relations, as Peet and Watts (2004) point out, requires that social workers pay attention to non-local power relations as well.

CONCLUSION

In approaching a rural, regional or remote community, social workers are called on to have a broad analysis of the historical, social, economic, ecological and political background of a specific place. A place-based social work model draws on critical ecological systems theory as well as an anti-oppressive and empowerment perspective to pay attention to how power relations dynamically impact on various sub-groups in a 'community'. A sustainable livelihoods framework provides a tool for analysis that can be used discursively with community members, either informally or through a participatory action research approach in a more formal project setting, to develop an intercultural understanding of the specific location and livelihood strategies. This approach to working with rural, regional and remote communities highlights the contextual nature of social work practice more generally. The role of generic social workers needs to include research as an important mode of social work practice. The emphasis on context highlights the necessity of sound policy analysis skills in critically appraising governmental directions and the likely effects on 'target populations' or geographic locations of policies, especially on places where residents draw on natural resources for livelihoods strategies.

RECOMMENDED READING

Lockie, S. & Bourke, L. (2001) *Rurality Bites*. Pluto Press, Sydney.

Rural Society Journal, journal of global research into rural social problems and sustainable communities, School of Humanities and Social Sciences, Charles Sturt University, Wagga Wagga, NSW.

Shaw, M. (2008) Community development and the politics of community. *Community Development Journal*, 43(1), 24–36.

Simpson, M.C. (2009) An integrated approach to assess the impacts of tourism on community development and sustainable livelihoods. *Community Development Journal*, 44(2), 186–208.

Zapf, M.K. (2009) *Social Work and the Environment: Understanding people and place*. Canadian Scholars' Press, Toronto.

3

COLLABORATING
WITHIN AND ACROSS
INTERPROFESSIONAL TEAMS

Liz Beddoe and Mollie Burley

CHAPTER OBJECTIVES

- To discuss the principles for successful interprofessional team-work and consider how these relationships can be formed and developed over time.
- To provide examples of how social workers make constructive contributions to interprofessional teams in different contexts.
- To examine some of the challenges for maintaining interprofessional relationships.
- To identify strategies for strengthening teamwork, ongoing learning and development for social workers in rural practice.

INTRODUCTION

Well-developed communication skills facilitate effective work with both colleagues and members of other professions, and are thus a core element of effective social work in any setting. Collaborating with other disciplines to provide service to client groups and meet agency objectives is vital for safe work in rural communities.

INTERPROFESSIONAL COLLABORATION

Interprofessional collaborative practice is believed to be a key strategy to enhance quality client-centred service delivery and excellent communication. The literature of recent decades has drawn our attention to the ways in which specific disciplines have tended to work within silos, isolated from each other and sometimes clashing, through lack of good communication. This way of working greatly limits the collaborative style needed to address complex health and social issues effectively.

CASE STUDY: A PROBLEM SHARED

Carole works as a social worker in community health in a very small country town. Malia is a nurse in the same service and is providing post-operative wound care for Juliet (aged nine), who has had recent abdominal surgery. A treatment plan was provided by the surgical registrar at the hospital and Juliet is due to go back in for a check-up in ten days' time. Juliet's mother Linda is having chemotherapy, which means being away for a week at a time. Her father Joe has suffered from depression, and is close to his coping limits. The family is fairly isolated with limited input from extended family, who live interstate. There is a 120-kilometre drive to the hospital where both Linda and Juliet are patients. On a home visit, Carole finds Juliet in a miserable state; her wound is infected and she is complaining of pain. Carole wants someone to take Juliet back to the surgical clinic early but the family is on a very limited budget and Joe is adamant he wants to wait until Linda's appointment in a week rather than make two trips. Carole feels that this family is really vulnerable and is particularly worried about Juliet's health. She and Malia set up a meeting with Timothy, the family's GP. After some animated discussion, the group is able to focus on a sensible plan to support the family.

Reflective questions

- What do you think might be the main elements of the discussion?
- What might be the power dynamics operating in this discussion?
- What differences might influence the three professionals in their approaches to Juliet's family?
- Who else might need to be called in to offer help or provide intervention?
- What would make this group of professionals a team rather than just colleagues?

The case study and reflective questions above point to some of the challenges of working in multidisciplinary teams anywhere. We know from experience that different professionals may have particular ways of seeing (and acting in) the world. Often this is a benefit for clients, as each professional brings their own expertise and knowledge to bear on problems. But sometimes these differences in perspective can cause tension and conflict. Hugh G. Petrie (1976, cited in Hall, 2005: 190) suggests that professional practitioners develop a cognitive map during their training and practice where personal characteristics and experience, together with individual and professional values and beliefs, determine some key aspects of their practice.

In rural practice, the risks of isolation are greater but the benefits of excellent teamwork are even more significant. When practitioners have been raised in a rural area, their perspective is attuned to rural life and work, assisting a smooth transition into their professional life. However, if practitioners are from an urban setting, another part of the country or overseas, understanding the differences between rural and urban will require some adjustment of both their way of working and their cognitive map. Professional values emphasise aspects of working with service users differently: in some professions, science rules decision-making and interaction; in others, listening to client stories is the mode of intervention most valued. Language is often an important means of differentiation (Hall, 2005). Working in rural communities creates opportunities to safely reduce professional distance and to work with a range of different disciplines, bringing together knowledge distilled from research, teaching and practice wisdom.

Interprofessional work involves three important aspects: an understanding of both service user and professional experiences and contexts; clarity about different professional perspectives, theory and policies; and creative and committed joint work to find solutions to problems identified (Smith & Anderson, 2008: 769).

As a result of strong lobbying, Australia has begun to give more recognition to the urban–rural differences in service delivery, and specific rural policy development has become a reality. The National Rural Health Alliance (NRHA), with 31 member organisations, has significant influence at a government policy level (NRHA, 2011). The NRHA has maintained pressure on the federal government to focus on rural issues. Good examples of this impetus are the development of alternative rural service models—programs that support rural and remote clients' access to metropolitan specialist services, and programs that provide training and support for rural health and social welfare practitioners. In Australia, the 2010 Gillard federal election win was attributed to support from three rural independent members of parliament. These members argued strongly for their 'rural constituencies', and as a result all government policy is now to be tested for 'rural appropriateness and applicability', supporting the recognition that one policy does not fit all situations (Gillard et al., 2010: Appendix B).

The development of strong policy initiatives for greater collaboration in rural services is not confined to Australia. Around the world, major research and policy development has addressed the increasingly complex health and social care needs of diverse communities. In rural and remote settings, patient safety, staff shortages and the challenges identified by Christiane Brems and colleagues (2006) mean that social workers, police, corrections officers, social welfare workers and health practitioners must be able to work collaboratively across their professional boundaries. Multi-professional networks ensure consistent, continuous and reliable service delivery. Networks—both formal and informal—are essential in rural practice as practitioners face situations that may require expertise beyond their level of skill or experience. One example from a small rural community is the challenge posed for a key professional when working with an aggressive/violent client who is unwell with a mental health disorder. Immediate assistance and support would be required during such a crisis. In this example, an interprofessional team (actual or virtual) would work together to support the local practitioner and to assist the client in their recovery. In such a situation, a social work practitioner might work alongside individuals who are members of the voluntary Country Fire Authority and State Emergency Services, volunteer ambulance officers, members of the Red Cross, members of the school parents' association and members of the football/cricket/netball club to support such clients during their everyday professional role. It is often these types of people/groups who respond during a crisis in rural communities, so building networks and relationships with a wide range of community groups and service providers is extremely important to establish the levels of trust and respect required to work together in a crisis.

Across the globe, initiatives to improve interprofessional collaborative practice have been on the policy agenda. The World Health Organization (WHO) has been a significant body in promoting interprofessional learning, and in 2010 released the *Framework for Action on Interprofessional Education and Collaborative Practice* report, which challenges health policy-makers to support the change to interprofessional collaboration. This new report (WHO, 2010) emphasises that research and experience have demonstrated that the team-based, or a collaborative, approach to health care is the best way forward, as clearly no single health discipline can provide the comprehensive service delivery needed for people with complex needs, whether in rural or urban areas (Australian Council for Safety and Quality in Health Care, 2005). The response to the Victorian bushfires of 2009 provides an example of how vital interprofessional teamwork is to rural communities.

CASE STUDY: RURAL VICTORIAN BUSHFIRES OF 2009

The tragedy that struck Victoria in the summer of 2009 was acknowledged around the world. Following devastating bush-fires, more than 100 people lost their lives, more than 1000 homes were destroyed or damaged and many thousands of people were dislocated from their homes. Once the initial emergency was under control, a vast number of organisa-tions came together to begin the recovery program. Led by the recently retired Police Commissioner, Christine Nixon, a recovery taskforce was formed to take stock of the situation, deal with immediate issues such as food, shelter and first aid, and implement a recovery program. Large sums donated for the victims were received from groups/clubs, the retail sector and private citizens from around Australia and the world. The fire-affected areas were searched for injured wildlife, with volunteers and vets seeking to treat and care for animals (you may recall the striking picture of a koala being given water to drink by a CFA volunteer).

While all this activity was apparent, out of the public eye the social workers, counsellors, psychologists, primary health workers, community and government services were working with the victims to assist them to deal with the impact of 'Black Saturday' on their lives. Two years after this tragic event occurred, we have been reminded that people involved in this emergency (victim, volunteer or service agency person-nel) who previously had appeared to be coping may find that they still require some assistance/support.

Reflective questions

- Which social welfare services would you expect to be involved in managing the immediate crisis?
- What role might they play?
- What strategies would you implement if you were asked to assist a victim of this crisis after the emergency is over?
- Who else/what other agencies could be called in to offer help or support immediately?
- What might the longer-term personal issues be for those helping professionals involved in responding to the immediate crisis?

While crisis work is particularly challenging, understanding how to work across professional boundaries is a vital component of rural social work. A brief exploration of some of the terminology of interprofessional work follows.

DEFINITIONAL ISSUES: INTERPROFESSIONAL WORK AND COLLABORATIVE WORK

Three kinds of practice in which different professions work together can be identified. Social workers will come across these terms in practice.

1 **Interprofessional practice (IPP).** There is no agreed specific definition for IPP; however, the term implies a broader understanding of the need to collaborate in practice. It is not specifically oriented to patient care and is driven by the agenda and context of the environment. There are expectations that professionals will act in this way.
2 **Interprofessional collaborative practice (IPC).** Interprofessional collaboration occurs when

two or more individuals from different backgrounds with complementary skills, interact to create a shared understanding that none had previously possessed or could have come to on their own. (WHO, 2010: 36)

45

3 **Transdisciplinary work.** A third kind of working together is identified in the newer term 'transdisciplinary', used to describe practice where one discipline extends its scope of practice into the area of another discipline. Examples include a limited range of remote X-ray operator radiography being conducted by licensed nurses or general practitioners. The definition is: 'where professionals undertake tasks outside their normal professional roles' (Oandasan & Reeves, 2005).

Whichever type of practice dominates, all have their origins in an international movement towards greater collaboration, accelerated by public and government concerns about vulnerable clients slipping through the net with great harm ensuing (Kemshall, 2010).

POLICY AND PRACTICE INFLUENCES: INTERNATIONAL AND AUSTRALIAN PERSPECTIVES

Policy on interprofessional work historically has been developed out of the need for systemic change, as identified in cases where outcomes have gone awry. In social work, social policy is often driven by the high-profile child abuse or mental health tragedies that receive much media attention and promote public anxiety (Kemshall, 2010). Two oft-cited international examples can be found in the United Kingdom, where the policy imperative for change was spurred by the death of Victoria Climbié and by the Bristol Infirmary Inquiry (Butler & Drakeford, 2005). Victoria Climbié was a young girl brought to the United Kingdom from France to live with her aunt with the intent of getting better housing. Over a number of years, Victoria was seen by up to eleven health and social care agencies and made numerous visits to hospital; yet, despite documentation indicating concern for her care, no firm steps were taken to protect her welfare. Ultimately, Victoria's state of ongoing neglect resulted in her death. The inquiry established to review this case indicated that a lack of communication between professionals had contributed to this outcome. The Bristol inquiry involved a hospital where the paediatric surgeons were conducting heart surgery over a number of years with very poor outcomes and consequent deaths of children. The surgical technique was not proven to be effective by research, yet the surgeons continued this treatment. Once again, an inquiry found that poor communication between all team members and medical dominance were features of the case (Butler & Drakeford, 2005).

Australia has not been immune to failures in duty of care, with two cases of particular note—that of Daniel Valerio in 1990, and more recently that of Dr Jayant Patel. Both failures have occurred as a result of a lack of interprofessional cooperation, collaboration and communication, and have resulted in changes to practice, policy and legislation. Aged just two years and four months, Daniel Valerio was battered to death by his stepfather. Policy-makers were shocked that 21 professionals had seen Daniel prior to his murder, includ-ing doctors and a teacher (Victorian Department of Community Services & Fogarty, 1991). The areas cited as causes of this failure of duty of care include poor management, staff shortages, failure to follow procedures, inadequate recording, role confusion and failure to communicate. One outcome of Daniel's death was a change in the law in 1993, which resulted in the implementation of mandatory reporting of suspected child abuse cases by police, doctors, nurses and teachers.

The second example is that of Dr Patel, who was accused of gross incompetence while working at Bundaberg Base Hospital in Queensland between 2003 and 2005. Various staff at the hospital had reported concerns about his clinical judgement, leading to some nurses hiding patients from him for their protection (BBC News, 2010). Public concern eventually forced two powerful inquiries, the Royal Commission investigating Dr Patel (Davies Inquiry) and the Queensland health system (Morris Inquiry). The outcomes of these two inquiries have resulted in significant changes in practice, policy and legislation.

Following on from a number of such cases in the second half of the last decade, policy changes have explored new models such as primary health care and interprofessional collaboration. Key issues driving policy change have focused on supporting workforce flex-ibility, reducing medical dominance and meeting consumer expecta-tions of increased involvement in decisions about care (Légaré et al., 2011). Additional drivers for policy change include:

- the impact of the ageing population
- progressive technological advances
- rising health-care costs
- increasing life expectancy
- reduction in the health-care workforce
- the need to address rural access to services (Haxton & Boelk, 2010: 527).

The desirability of interprofessional collaboration, particularly in the rural context, is evident in terms of sharing resources (transport, buildings, and communications technology) and reliance on teamwork between professionals where not all team members are co-located.

SAFETY AND ISOLATION: WORKING WITH COLLEAGUES FOR SAFETY

As noted in Chapter 1, there are numerous ways in which rural life is conceptualised: the rugged, gendered imagery or the romantic ideals of rural life are synonymous with a sense of community, a healthier lifestyle and idyllic locations. The alternative perspective is somewhat different, speaking of isolation and disenfranchisement—especially when we compare urban to rural populations and find that rural people may be less well served by health care and human services, especially for specialist input including hospice care (Haxton & Boelk, 2010). Some research has painted a picture of rural Australia in which family violence is problematic and often hidden (Wendt, 2009). Rural social work has often focused on the identification of the problems faced by practitioners, with a major emphasis on the importance of ongoing professional development, a work–life balance and careful management of professional and personal boundaries (Lonne & Cheers, 2004). Despite these professional challenges, work in rural locations should also be acknowledged for providing excellent opportunities for interprofessional collaboration and practice. Teams are usually smaller; members are well known to each other and tend to work across professional boundaries; the care provided is often more holistic than in larger teams, or in larger services; and workers can follow their client or patient through from admission to discharge from the service. A major advantage of rural practice is that it provides many opportunities to undertake shared visits/consultations with clients to facilitate joint assessment and intervention.

Practice in rural services frequently requires an understanding of different cultures, as health-care practitioners may work with Indigenous or Maori populations, and others, such as refugees from Africa or Asia. Each of these populations has its own specific health and cultural issues, so service delivery needs to be flexible, integrated, coordinated and delivered in a culturally secure environment by a team that includes experienced Indigenous health workers providing the link between these vulnerable communities and the health and welfare services (Spencer et al., 2010). A more in-depth examination of social work with diverse populations is offered in Chapter 10.

CONTRIBUTING TO MULTI-DISCIPLINARY TEAMWORK

This section explores the ways in which professional cultures can operate as barriers in teams. It is a well-reported view that interprofessional and interagency dynamics can hinder effective service delivery to users of health and social care services. Challenges to interprofessional collaboration include differing levels of perceived status and power; diverse knowledge and related terminology; varying focus; and different values and expectations of teamwork versus individual autonomy.

In social work, we do not need to be reminded how often miscommunication can cause problems in care and protection, justice and mental health (Stanley & Manthorpe, 2004). Poor communication is neither accidental nor deliberate; it develops through poorly managed systems, professional rivalries, status issues, territorial grey areas and stereotypical assumptions. All of these factors can impact negatively on how people work together. Pippa Hall (2005: 193) has suggested that the following six collaborative skills are essential for effective teamwork:

- cooperation
- assertiveness
- responsibility
- communication
- autonomy, and
- coordination.

These skills are tools that enable each professional to explore and understand their fellow team members' cognitive maps. Support for these elements is a fundamental requirement for all professionals. Trust and respect for a colleague is vital, as without these dispositions, interprofessional collaboration, cooperation and teamwork will be weakened or absent. Trust and respect need to be earned, beginning with an appreciation of each other's roles; the display of competency and capability (generally in shared decision-making) among team members; the development of shared goals focusing on client/patient-centred care; and knowledge of the community or

49

client/patient group. Working across boundaries—including those between professional disciplines, between agencies and organisations, and between professionals, community activists and volunteers—can provide powerful dynamics for positive change and creative solutions. Jessica E. Haxton and Amy Z. Boelk (2010: 546), for example, suggest that social workers can encourage local policy-makers and funders to bring 'together various constituencies in a community coalition . . . to address pervasive social issues'. A coalition of community leaders, health and social service professionals, members of NGOs, church groups and consumer groups can assemble a strong network that can help develop services and act as an effective advocate for policy change.

CASE STUDY: BUILDING NETWORKS FOR CHANGE

Mandy, a school-based social worker, notices lots of struggling parents in the group of mining towns in her region. The fathers are away from home on long shifts, and there are tensions with the mothers when they are home, mainly around parenting styles and money management. Mandy is seeing many stressed kids, a number of them with repeated bruising and other minor injuries. Mothers often report being exhausted and resentful. One day Mandy talks to a woman, Josie, who feels that a mothers' group might be a neutral way of introducing parenting skills in a community that prides itself on toughness and independence. Mandy and Josie team up with the enthusiastic local primary school principal and they agree that they will set something up. Mandy approaches the supportive town mayor, who in turn talks to a popular and respected local state MP. The MP arranges some funding to set up an informal action group. This group arranges not only to get a well-received parenting program to the community but also to get local women trained as peer-facilitators.

Reflections

- Think about the process of getting a steering group going to deliver a program. What do you think might be the important steps to take?
- Who else needs to be involved?
- Identify the skills Mandy will utilise in this project.

- What might be some of the obstacles Mandy could face along the way?
- How could you ensure some long-term change?

Social workers in rural settings encounter many social and health inequalities, and for rural practice to address these it is suggested that collaborative approaches are required (Whiteside, 2004). Brems and colleagues (2006) report that health-care providers in rural areas struggle more with resource limitations, confidentiality limitations, overlapping roles, provider travel, service access and training constraints as significant barriers to service delivery. They note that the smaller a provider's practice community, the greater the reports of obstacles, with the most severe issues reported in small rural communities (2006: 105). Addressing rural challenges effectively requires an approach that recognises all the assets within each community, including informal and formal sector input.

CHALLENGES TO TEAMWORK

Social work in any setting requires cooperation and information-sharing between health and community sector social workers and those working in statutory (mandated) practice. Child welfare services employ many social workers in rural settings, and these services face particular challenges. In everyday work, statutory (or mandated) services are interdependent on the relationships between providers of family support services, police and justice services and the primary health-care system. As noted above, there is a substantial agenda of work for primary care and social work to provide better health care and child protection (Marsh, 2006). Disputes in this area are often about thresholds of risk for children, but similar issues may apply regarding the needs of older people living alone, or the safety of people managing mental illness. A UK study found that difficulties between child protection and mental health services often focused on the different thresholds and codes of practice adopted by each profession, resulting in conflict around risk assessment (Barbour et al., 2002: 327–9). In such circumstances, conflict, role and boundary issues put desired outcomes for vulnerable service users at risk. Issues of power and organisational culture are not usually considered in detail in the policy-making sphere;

instead, 'there is an expectation that by decreeing that it will be so, collaboration will happen' (Beddoe & Davys, 2008: 40). There is broad consensus that power is a present and potent issue in both the relationships between professional and service users, and among the professionals themselves (Smith, 2008: 115).

As noted earlier in this chapter, differences in knowledge and training, with unacknowledged power differentials, can lead to tensions in multidisciplinary teams. Such conflict and rivalry are often grounded in the history of the development of different professions. Hall (2005: 190), describing the evolution of the health professions, suggests:

> Each profession has struggled to define its identity, values, sphere of practice and role in patient care. This has led to each health care profession working within its own silo to ensure its members . . . have common experiences, values, approaches to problem-solving and language for professional tools.

During their initial professional education, those in each occupational group not only learn the essential knowledge and skills for the practice of their profession, but also become socialised into the values and norms of their vocation. Pippa Hall and Lynda Weaver (2001) suggest that each profession might attract people with different and distinctive learning styles and approaches to problems; this in turn affects communication. Each profession has a different culture, which includes values, beliefs, attitudes, customs and behaviours. We value—and indeed exclaim—our differences as vital to our sense of professional identity, but there is a 'dark side' to these identities. If differences produce territorial disputes, conflict can challenge how well we work together.

As described earlier in the chapter, governments have in recent decades worked with social services and health-care systems to reduce the problems that can result if communication is affected by territorial problems. Roger Smith and Liz Anderson (2008) attribute the drive for change to a number of factors: the 'increasing sense of interdependency arising from the recognition of the holistic nature of needs'; the challenges of working in complex systems; the influence of systems and ecological perspectives; and the recognition of the rights of service users, which 'whether driven by consumerist ideas or principles of social justice, required the development of responses which crossed arbitrary organisational boundaries' (2008: 760–1).

In rural communities, the social services, emergency services and health-care system need to cooperate for many practical reasons, so rigid boundaries are neither feasible nor desirable. These groups rarely come together for regular meetings, so it is important to make and take opportunities to engage with other rural service providers and to discuss how best to work together. Some communities undertake 'hypothetical' exercises where they practise managing emergency responses, but it is the everyday occurrences that also require practice—and opportunities to enhance everyday communication strategies can be very limited. Given physical distances, social complexity and the particular challenges of rural and remote areas, teamwork must span boundaries.

CLINICAL DECISION-MAKING

A major component of successful teamwork is effective clinical decision-making. How decisions are made is not easily articulated by experienced practitioners, since many occur unconsciously as practitioners consider the potential issues involved in a specific case. Clinical reasoning or decision-making is defined as a 'process of reflective understanding of the clinical problem, in order to provide a sound basis for clinical intervention' (Higgs & Jones, 2000: 10). Elizabeth Quinlan and Susan Robertson (2010: 573) found that 'mutual understanding between team members ebbs and flows over the course of their collective clinical decisions', within which different professional knowledge is exchanged in the context of teams 'producing new knowledge'. Furthermore, 'as the extent of mutual understanding within the team increases, decision making becomes more equally shared among team members' (2010: 565). They also suggest that 'greater mutual understanding is achieved under the ideal circumstances of team members coming to clinical decisions with high levels of knowledge, with a well-developed discourse ethic, and with little or no occupational distance between them' (2010: 568).

Of course, individuals, families and even communities have the right to be involved in decisions about the outcomes of professional intervention. In a recent article, France Légaré and colleagues (2011: 20–2) presented a new model of shared decision-making designed to promote an interprofessional collaborative approach. They describe steps in the decision-making process as occurring at the micro, meso and macro levels. At the micro level, there are six steps involved in facilitating shared decision-making:

1 Professionals share their knowledge and understanding of the options with the patient.
2 Information is exchanged about the potential benefits and harms of the options.
3 Values clarification is carried out by all those involved in the decision-making process.
4 The feasibility of the options is considered.
5 Actual decision. With the practitioners' help, the service user identifies the preferred option. Experts in this model share their preference with the patient in the form of a recommendation.
6 The service users are supported to ensure that the options chosen have a favourable outcome. There is a need to evaluate whether the implementation goes ahead as planned. (Légaré et al., 2011: 20–1)

In this model, the meso level acknowledges the different individual team member roles and at the macro level there is an examination of factors from the health and care systems and 'global environmental elements such as resources, government policies, cultural values, professional organisations and rules' that have the capacity to influence 'how the team is organised and functions' (Légaré et al., 2011: 21).

Reflective questions

- How well does this model translate into a rural health and social service environment?
- Does this model fit well alongside social work approaches such as family decision-making conferencing?
- What sort of strategies might be used to evaluate interpersonal collaborative decision-making in rural services?

All good practice is underpinned by effective, career-long professional supervision and continuing education. In the final section of this chapter, we explore the challenges and opportunities afforded by rural practice. Ongoing learning in professional practice often centres around the needs of people who share 'a concern, a set of problems, or a passion about a topic, and who deepen their knowledge and expertise in this area by interacting on an ongoing basis' (Wenger et al., 2002: 4). The challenge of rural practice is to enable such interactions to occur.

INTERPROFESSIONAL LEARNING AND ICT

Interprofessional learning is one major strategy adopted to meet the challenges of improved collaboration between disciplines, but this approach is mainly confined to public health and government social agencies, which often have common administrative systems. In rural settings, these complex bureaucracies may be in microcosm, and even with modern technology, 'on-the-ground' communication is essential. Education providers and employers with budget constraints have embraced a range of technologies to deliver courses, facilitate skills acquisition, and support assessment, diagnosis and clinical decision-making at the coalface. Distance education programs using videoconferencing have facilitated the development of rural professional education and have provided greater access for international students. In addition, continuing professional development activities can effectively be supported, using distance modes, in rural environments where distance may prevent easy access or when resources are severely limited.

In health, telemedicine has also provided much-needed support for small rural health-care agencies, providing the means for staff to network for consultation and examination and discuss treatment recommendations. E-learning technologies (new software, online education, DVDs, media players, the internet, blogs, social networking sites and SMS reminders) offer a mixed approach to education and practice that is stimulating and engaging for learners, facilitates collaborative activities and supports the development of appropriate knowledge-management skills (Williams & Lakhani, 2010). Keith Brownlee and colleagues (2010: 630) found in a study of technology in Canadian rural social work that resource and geographical challenges such as professional isolation, training, supervision, scarcity of resources and limited professional expertise were 'regularly identified by participants as areas in which communications technology had positively impacted on service delivery'.

While all this technology sounds wonderful, there are significant barriers to implementation, with gaps existing between what is currently available and what is required to develop future practice. These barriers exist in relation to infrastructure, workers trained in these practices, skilled and reliable technical training and support staff, and potential concerns about privacy and security of client data. More significantly, technologies do not necessarily address the biggest challenges faced by rural social workers. Brownlee and colleagues observed in their Canadian research that there was no indication from social workers that technology had been used to address the issues of relationship-building and dual relationships:

> Many social workers reported that northern [rural] communities, for now, still preferred personal, face-to-face contact. The relationship they established with a worker, and the familiarity of that relationship, seemed to be precursors to developing trust and accessing services. (2010: 631)

Access to ongoing supervision is an important element of continuing education for rural social workers. Clinical supervision is mandatory for social workers and many other health professionals, and a number of models exist for delivering supervision. Junior staff may undertake clinical supervision with a more senior member of the agency's staff while more senior practitioners usually undertake external supervision face to face or via the telephone. While some professions may insist on *intra*professional supervision, interprofessional supervision can provide excellent support for safe and growing practice, especially where face-to-face contact is so important in terms of establishing trust and respect. Opportunities for interprofessional learning and supervision should be embraced, as they provide confirmation of the things held in common among disciplines and build respect for the differences that make each professional contribution unique. 'Learning to focus on relationships and mutuality rather than knowledge from and for specific clinical domains is potentially transformative' (Beddoe & Davys, 2008: 40).

In rural areas, practitioners may often need to be creative when looking for supervision. Hugh Crago and Margo Crago (2002) discuss the complaint 'But you can't get good supervision in the country' and suggest a number of options, with ideas for how best to set these up. Peer supervision within agencies or among a group of agencies is a good option and often relatively inexpensive. Peer and group supervision may also utilise the expertise of a wider range of disciplines. While social workers will need to have some social work supervision to meet AASW requirements, for someone who is the only child health social worker in the region, supervision with an excellent nurse practitioner in the field might be very satisfying. Group and peer approaches to supervision are also beneficial, as they will expand the skill base for supervision in the community. Email and social networking sites also provide an effective medium for maintaining contact with peers, enabling the professional networks established in social work training to remain an active and vital part of the professional infrastructure for a 'networked' rural social worker.

SUMMARY

This chapter has emphasised effective teamwork and relationship-building as crucial to safe practice in rural contexts. Social work in rural practice can be challenging, but holding a strong sense of professional identity while being a generous member of an interprofessional team can outweigh the barriers or deficits. Viewing other professionals, community experts and informal networks as a rich source of ideas, wisdom and support is an essential disposition. As you approach rural practice, whether as a student or a worker in a new job, make a plan to locate people who can engage in a mutually beneficial network. If resources seem thin on the ground, use your community-development skills to innovate.

RECOMMENDED READING

Hammick, M., Freeth, D., Copperman, J. and Goodsman, D. (2009) *Being Interprofessional*. Polity Press, Cambridge, UK.

Meads, G. and Ashcroft, J., with Barr, H., Scott, R. and Wild, A. (2005) *The Case for Interprofessional Collaboration: In health and social care*. CAIPE. Blackwell Publishing, Oxford.

PART III

Fields of practice in rural settings

4

SECURING AFFORDABLE
HOUSING IN RURAL AND
REMOTE TOWNS

Uschi Bay with Yvonne Jenkins

CHAPTER OBJECTIVES

- To outline the current national housing issues and research on affordability and availability of housing in regional, rural and remote Australia.
- To highlight how livelihood changes—like the resources boom and the sea- and tree-change movements—have impacted on housing affordability in remote, rural and regional towns.
- To explore alternative rental housing options that can provide security of tenure, involvement in decision-making about tenancy issues and the maintenance of properties.

INTRODUCTION

It is becoming more difficult to secure affordable housing in Australia, not only in cities but also in regional and rural towns—especially for families on only one income, or on lower to medium incomes. The great Australian dream has been to buy and own a house, even though this used to take many wage earners most of their working lives to achieve. Now, however, the dream of home ownership has become unaffordable for many people, as house prices have increased fivefold over the last two decades while wages have merely doubled. It now takes two solid incomes and a sizeable deposit or savings to afford a house in many areas. House prices can seem more affordable in some rural and regional centres, but the overall cost of living, including access to public transport, education, child care and health care, combined with fewer employment opportunities and lower pay rates, makes such a move both difficult and costly. Alternative policies and models of housing may offer hope to the over one million people in Australia who are currently suffering the effects of housing stress, inadequate housing or homelessness.

It is common knowledge that house prices have soared over the last few decades in major metropolitan cities, especially Sydney, Perth and Melbourne. A significant gap between those people who are homeowners and those who are renting has developed, with many families finding it difficult to obtain secure and affordable rental accommodation or to be able to purchase a home over the longer term. In major cities, many low-income people are being forced out, to 'the far-flung outer suburbs, where you have no social support or networks' (Shaw, 2011: 7). This situation is creating significant housing stress for people who are not already homeowners, and a wealth gap between those who own their homes or are paying off a mortgage and those in rental accommodation. Many Australians are likely to find they are 'trapped in private rental housing' (Beer et al., 2011: 2) and younger people are expected to find it extremely difficult to buy into the housing sector without assistance from their families. It is predicted that 'by 2020, something like 40 per cent of Australians will be long-term or permanent renters' (Burke, cited in Edwards, 2011: 3).

There is limited research into rural, regional and remote housing, but recent publications indicate that 'housing affordability is a major challenge for particular groups in rural and regional Australia' (Beer et al., 2011: 2). From an anti-oppressive and empowerment perspective, these housing gaps and the significant pressure being faced particularly by younger, older, Aboriginal and low-income people when it comes to finding housing in rural, regional and remote areas is a serious issue that needs to be tackled by social workers. We will highlight the specific housing issues in resource boom towns and sea- and tree-change locations to highlight the impact of geography and livelihoods on various sub-groups in these locations.

There is a perception that public, community and social housing is not needed or is not in demand in rural and regional areas, and the 2009 federal government Stimulus Package did not include funding for many such settlements. Social housing can only be provided for those who are in highest need, yet the biggest unmet demand for housing stock comes from people on low to medium incomes (Beer ct al., 2011). Social workers can contribute to addressing these housing issues through researching local trends closely and convening local, regional, state or national housing networks to collate data. They can take action with communities by advocating for service development, by disseminating information on housing programs and schemes to rural, regional and remote communities, and by assisting with grant and tender writing.

There is an opportunity for social workers to contribute to these changes through the development of an understanding of how 'the geography of housing affordability and unaffordability is highly variable' within and between the diverse settlement types in Australia (Beer et al., 2011: 2). Different factors impinge on diverse settlements such as resource boom towns, coastal sea-change and tree-change destinations, Aboriginal homelands in desert Australia, agriculturally based country towns and hinterlands in relation to housing opportunities and livelihood strategies. We will outline some of these factors in this chapter, and also explore alternate housing options and strategies that aim to ensure low-income people, older people and younger people, people with disabilities and Aboriginal people 'can live in housing with the same security and dignity as owners' (Burke, cited in Edwards, 2011: 3).

HOUSING AFFORDABILITY CRISIS

Housing affordability is linked to the amount of household income required to provide shelter to a family or single person. When housing costs take up more than 30 per cent of a household's income, that household is considered to be experiencing housing stress. It is argued that a better measure of housing stress is the ratio of earnings to house prices (Beer et al., 2011). As rental rates are linked to house prices, this applies both to households that comprise owner-occupiers making mortgage repayments and to households paying rent. In Australia, between 1980 and 2002 the basic wage (after tax) rose 300 per cent, but the median house price rose 600 per cent (Wilkinson, 2005: 32). According to National Shelter, the peak advocacy group on housing issues in Australia, two of the key measures of the housing crisis are the shortage of private rental dwellings that are available and affordable to low- and lower-income people, and the number of people on waiting lists for social housing and the number of homeless people on

Census night. In 2007–08, there was a shortage of nearly half a million available and affordable private rental dwellings, with nearly 200 000 of these being in regional, rural and remote locations. 'There were 248,419 applicants waiting for social housing in Australia in 2010. On census night in 2006, there were 105,000 homeless people in Australia' (National Shelter, 2011).

The current crisis in housing affordability is particularly dire for those people not considered to be in sufficient need or on a low enough income to attain social housing, and who have to compete in the increasingly competitive private rental market. Even if people gain Commonwealth Rental Assistance, the 'cheapest rents in many regional towns are out of reach of many low-income families and such families are often outbid or excluded due to their household characteristics' (Beer et al., 2011: 3). Discrimination against young people, or families with children, or on the basis of race or sexual orientation is common in the rental market (Beer et al., 2011).

The short supply of affordable rental housing is impacting upon low-income families and 'plunging families reliant on government benefits into serious rental stress' (Kell, cited in Horin, 2011: 52). 'Moving to a cheaper area sounds like a solution but these families often can't afford the relocation costs and where rent is cheaper, unemployment is often higher' (Kell, cited in Horin, 2011: 52). It is a 'common assumption that housing outside the capitals is more affordable' (Beer et al., 2011: 18). There are other costs involved in relocating to the fringes of cities, regional towns or more remote locations. Access to health care, education, child care and public transport services is often more costly, or is simply not locally available. Long commutes to work can place additional stress on families, especially those with young children. In addition, recent research indicates that the 'incidence of housing stress among tenants in rural and regional centres is [as] acute as in the major metropolitan centres' (Beer et al., 2011: 2).

In rural, remote and regional settlements, there are various significant impediments to housing supply, both for the private rental market and home ownership. There are complex links to livelihood strategies, natural amenities and the availability of land in many areas that contribute to the low levels of housing availability. This shortage of available and affordable housing impacts on labour market shortages, especially for essential workers like teachers, nurses, social workers and other service providers. The lack of experienced social housing landlords who can manage this type of program in rural and remote settings can also mean that this housing option is not readily available to low-income or differently abled people, or to older and younger age groups. Often the lack of services means that these groups feel 'that they are forced to leave their region in order to secure services in a larger regional centre' (Beer et al., 2011: 6).

The costs of land, size of land, planning rules and costs of linking amenities to land for residential development can make private developers and investors reluctant to invest in housing in various rural, regional and remote areas. 'Housing markets are not static and there are many types of housing markets evident across the landscape' in Australia (Beer et al., 2011: 30). Due to the diversity of the issues and the complexity, it is useful to take a place-based approach to exploring these housing issues further by focusing in this instance on resource boom towns and sea- and tree-change destinations.

RESOURCE BOOM TOWNS

Employment-led population growth impacts on relatively small towns when mines are opened or a resources boom occurs, suddenly driving the cost of housing extremely high. When demand exceeds supply and the income of mine workers far exceeds the income of locals, many residents find that their rents or rates become too high, and housing becomes unaffordable. In Port Hedland, Matthew Carney (2008) interviewed an Aboriginal man locally employed by the council for many years whose rent had become unaffordable; as a result, he was considering leaving his home town and his job to find more affordable housing. Local businesses indicated that they found it difficult to compete with the high wages paid by the mine to attract and retain workers. The ongoing in-migration of people from around Australia looking to work in the mines meant that there was a waiting list for housing even at the caravan park, and that the cost of even very basic housing became excessively high. Often the in-migrating workers had also been displaced by the high costs of housing in other areas of Australia, and were hoping to gain or regain a foothold in the housing market after a few years of working at the mines.

Sometimes mining companies find it difficult to house their workers. In these instances, they use fly-in/fly-out (FIFO) arrangements, where men generally leave their families in other parts of Australia to work a few weeks on and a few weeks off at the mine.

Sometimes mining companies provide barracks-style accommodation for their workers while working on site. Concern has been expressed by local residents about the kind of culture that is established in these places, and the way the workers use the town's amenities for recreation. More specifically, high levels of alcohol consumption and associated violence are particularly troubling. The lack of positive involvement by FIFO workers in the community, through activities like coaching sporting teams, is also regarded by locals as a lack of commitment to their small communities. Local governments and service agencies do find it difficult to provide consistent services to these types of communities, due to uncertainty of demand and the ever-changing numbers in the local population.

The shortage of available and affordable housing is often exacerbated by the slow release of land. At times, local land is owned by mining companies or by state governments. Both parties tend to be slow to respond to market indicators, and at times native title and nature-based environmental concerns also slow the availability of land for housing. These hurdles to providing affordable housing are linked to the livelihood strategies of various sub-groups in the community, and often the stock of publicly owned housing in such places is limited or inadequate. Further, because low-income people are not eligible for this housing, the gap between those who can afford exorbitant rent or mortgage rates and those who cannot creates serious levels of disadvantage. For instance, Fiona Haslam McKenzie and colleagues (2009) detail 'the resource industries' impact on the housing market of Karratha where prices and rents were forced up to levels well in excess of $800 000 [for a house] and $1000 a week [in rent]' (cited in Beer et al., 2011: 15). Similar effects of displacing low-income households to surrounding towns is also in evidence in coastal settlements.

SEA- AND TREE-CHANGE DESTINATIONS

The movement widely referred to as sea-change or tree-change involves people moving from city locations to regional and rural places that offer more affordable housing, as well as geographical and natural amenities like beaches or forests. Some more affluent people elect to move to coastal or forested places to cash in on the higher prices available for selling their inner-city properties. However, employment and education opportunities are less available, and commuting to work often means heavy reliance on cars, due to

inadequate or unavailable public transport. Over time, these conditions can make the move more expensive than anticipated:

> Land values in many coastal areas have risen dramatically in recent
> years and levels of housing stress in some coastal areas now exceed
> that experienced in some of the major capitals. This is occurring in
> a context of high levels of socio-economic disadvantage with many
> non-metropolitan coastal communities characterised by high propor-
> tions of low-income households and unemployment. (Squires &
> Gurran, 2005: 1)

The in-migration of older people to coastal settlements for their
retirement is also impacting on displacement of local people from their
housing in sea- or tree-change locations. The accompanying increases
in house prices and associated council rates mean that long-term residents can no longer afford to stay living in their houses. Many are
forced to move to the fringes of coastal towns, with inadequate public
transport, shopping, social and health services, further marginalising
older and low-income people in these locations.

Constraints on land availability for affordable housing are at times
impacted by environmental concerns, such as restrictions related to
flood plains, coastal erosion and sea inundation. Some of these
environmental aspects are expected to increase with climate change,
meaning that housing developments need to take into consideration
land use in relation to severe storms, high tides, road flooding and
landslides. Water supply is also an issue in many coastal communities. Visitors to these areas are not always aware that their activities
result in major depletion of water for the local residents.

In several coastal locations, workers supporting the local residents
and tourists cannot afford to rent or buy a house, and are forced
to commute from outlying towns. Often there is little or no public
transport available, and the costs of running a car can be an additional barrier to accessing work for low-income workers.

Despite there being a housing shortage, many houses are empty
for most of the year due to high levels of holiday home ownership
in sea- and tree-change locations. For instance, research undertaken
on the Mid-North Coast of New South Wales found that, despite
a desperate need for housing, more than 8000 homes were empty
(Cartwright, 2006: 3). High rates of non-permanent residents have
implications for securing funding for ongoing education, health and
other social services in these areas. Availability of human capital to

bid for community housing is limited, even if the local community supports such developments. At times rural and remote communities are reluctant to consider community housing (Beer et al., 2011).

HOUSING AFFORDABILITY FACTORS

Many regional centres experience sudden 'demand shocks' that can increase the cost of housing and create additional housing stress. For instance, temporary workers like a road crew working on a highway can push rental prices higher. The influx of university students or tourists into a regional town can exacerbate the rental market, and price rises remain inflated even after the workers, tourists or students leave. Long-term renters are disadvantaged by these changes, and many are forced into 'non-standard forms of accommodation such as garages or caravans' (Beer et al., 2011: 22).

In some regional areas, people are largely reliant on statutory incomes, and wages from paid employment are markedly lower in remote and rural areas. Paid work is often seasonal, casual and temporary, reinforcing the insecure and low levels of income. In such circumstances, families can easily fall behind in their rental payments and can find themselves insecure in the rental housing market.

Housing for older people is limited in some regional, rural and remote settings, and opportunities to downsize may not exist. Ageing in place may not be possible and older people are out-migrating off farms and from coastal settlements to larger regional centres especially as their health needs increase (Cartwright, 2006).

The limited supply of publicly owned dwellings is one factor that influences affordability of rental housing in regional, rural and remote locations. Much of the public housing stock when it was available has been sold off, and the remaining stock is usually older and less suitable, especially for people with special needs. The waiting lists for public housing are long and many people who are eligible are not bothering to register (Beer et al., 2011). There appears to be a lack of appreciation of housing needs in rural and remote areas by policy-makers located at a distance in more urban settings.

GOVERNMENT HOUSING POLICY

Government policies have a critical role to play in rural, remote and regional housing, and the impact of these policies over time has at times been positive, negative or both (Beer et al., 2011: 23). This is not the first time Australia has faced a major housing affordability and availability crisis. Following World War II, the federal government committed to a massive housing building program to increase desperately needed housing stock, rid the cities of slums and stimulate economic expansion. Most of the housing built under these programs was then sold off into private ownership and the housing that was left became public housing rental stock (Hayward, 1996).

The nomenclature in housing policy is confusing, and terms like social housing, community housing and public housing are often used interchangeably. It may be useful to point out that social housing is the umbrella term for all the government housing programs in Australia. Social housing comprises various programs: public rental housing, mainstream community housing, state-owned and managed Indigenous housing, the Crisis Accommodation Program (CAP) and Indigenous community housing (AIHW, 2010b). Public rental housing is publicly owned indirectly by all and administered by state and territory governments. Mainstream community housing is managed by not-for-profit organisations like churches, welfare organisations and community groups, which provide short-, medium- and long-term housing to low-income individuals. Crisis accommodation 'provides dwellings for use by government, churches and welfare organisations to provide assistance to people experiencing homelessness or imminent crisis' (AIHW 2010b: 2). Indigenous community housing consists of government-owned dwellings, which are managed by community housing organisations for Indigenous tenants.

The Chifley ALP-led federal government loaned money in 1945 to the state governments at low interest rates to assist in building homes for low-income earners. This housing was only available for rent, and the rental was charged at 20 per cent or one-fifth of the basic wage (Wilkinson, 2005: 6). To address housing affordability, it was then Labor Party policy to provide a 'good, cheap house, either for rent or purchase for people earning around the basic wage' (Barry, 1989: 278).

The role of government in providing housing to low-income earners changed with the new agreement between the federal government and the states in 1978. The Fraser Coalition government shifted the emphasis away from public housing to residual welfare housing by making public housing available only 'for those on pensions, unemployment benefits or disability payments' (Wilkinson, 2005:

18). Australian housing policy thus has focused on providing for the poorest and most disadvantaged people (66 per cent of public housing in 2008–09 was allocated to those in 'greatest need') (AIHW 2010b).

Community housing began in the 1980s and was considered a temporary scheme for people waiting for public housing (Wilkinson, 2005: 38). In 1995, the then Labor premier of New South Wales, Bob Carr, offered community housing as an alternative to public housing. Government-owned properties would be transferred to community housing associations to manage. This move was part of a broad shift in the way governments began to understand their responsibilities, by articulating the desire to set policy direction and not to be involved in the owning or delivery of housing services. Indeed, since the 1980s, governments in Australia have not intervened when house prices have risen steeply and wage increases have increased only slowly. In fact, governments have used microeconomic reform to restrain wage increases during this recent period of rapid house-price and rental-cost increases (see Wilkinson, 2005).

Recent policy innovations to address the affordability of housing in Australia have included the National Affordable Housing Agree-ment (NAHA) and the National Rental Affordability Scheme (NRAS). Andrew Beer and colleagues' (2011) recent research, includ-ing interviews with key stakeholders in various rural, regional and remote settlements, indicates that these schemes are not well known. The uptake of these options outside metropolitan regions relates to the absence of community organisations and investor resources, as well as the expertise needed to develop such initiatives. Developing housing programs of this order requires skills in calculating invest-ment risk, promoting institutional and human capital and collection of accurate demographic data, as well as substantial expertise in applying for funding and developing partnerships, and experience in managing housing stock and tenancy arrangements. A key role may exist here for social workers to address housing shortages through the process of bringing together people with the required knowledge and skills to work on housing in these particular locations.

There are now many different types of community housing organ-isations across Australia. Beer et al. (2011) point out that one of the issues in rural, remote and regional areas is that experienced commu-nity housing organisations are needed to apply for and manage new government housing projects under various housing affordability schemes. Many not-for-profit community housing organisations help to house people who belong to specific groups, such as single mothers, single elderly women and people with disabilities. One of the options governments have identified as a positive option for low-income people is rental housing cooperatives. Governments will sometimes provide funds to cooperatives to assist with the acquisition of housing. Rental cooperatives are required to adopt policies and procedures that are consistent and compliant with the National Community Housing Standards. The rental cooperatives are set up so that tenants pay the same rents as public tenants.

RENTAL HOUSING COOPERATIVES

Cooperative housing is rental housing for people on low to moderate incomes where members select tenants and manage and maintain the housing. This scheme provides long-term, secure and affordable housing. The government funds the building or purchase of dwellings, and the cooperative then self-manages these, making it a cost-effective alternative to other forms of social housing. Rents are used to cover running costs, upgrades, administration and training. Currently, there are around 50 rental housing cooperatives in urban and rural areas in New South Wales, with between five and 30 dwellings per cooperative. Some cooperatives are located in one building while others include separate houses within one suburb. Some cooperatives are rural, and houses are in clusters or spread throughout a town.

In Victoria, a modified cooperative housing model is being offered that is 'an alternative to the standard choice of renting or buying a home, by creating a rent-to-buy option for people who are otherwise locked out of the market' (Robertson, 2011: 10). The non-profit organisation working on this project is Common Equity Housing, which aims to assist people with incomes of up to $50 000 initially to rent the property at a rate capped at 75 per cent of the rental market; when their income improves, there is an option to buy the house or to move on. The project provides secure tenure and the opportunity for low-income earners to be involved in the maintenance of the property. Common Equity Housing is particularly interested in providing homes for young teachers and nurses: 'There are long-term benefits from staying in one place for a long time [rare when renting]; you get involved in social clubs in the area, you get involved in schools, just get to know people . . .' (Robertson, 2011: 10). Funding for this new project was approved under the federal National Rental Affordability Scheme.

Rental housing cooperatives are encouraged to meet local need and to specify the different types of people on low to moderate incomes who are to benefit from the housing, such as families, single people, young people, older people, people with special needs or people from diverse ethnic backgrounds. The following case study outlines how a group of local people in a small rural town set up a rental housing cooperative with the initial assistance of a social science student undertaking a social welfare field placement at a local Neighbourhood House.

CASE STUDY: DEVELOPING A RURAL HOUSING COOPERATIVE

A social science student undertaking a field placement was asked to research the availability of secure affordable rental housing in a local shire and to identify any gaps. As in many small towns, rental availability was limited, and the study revealed a major gap in availability of affordable rental properties and in security of tenure. The Neighbourhood House coordinator then invited local people to form a committee to write a submission for funding to set up a local housing cooperative. This committee met and expressed interest in acquiring housing under what was then called the New South Wales Common Equity Rental Cooperative Program.

The advantage of acquiring this type of housing is that cooperative members who will live in the houses have more control over the types of homes in which they live, as they are involved in the property selection and/or design for building new housing. The cooperative members' involvement is to ensure that the housing meets local community members' needs. However, the process of forming a rental housing cooperative is complex and daunting, especially for inexperienced people. One of the requirements for proceeding with a submission was gaining auspice from an incorporated body to be able to receive government funds. The Neighbourhood House auspiced the rental housing cooperative until it was incorporated and registered with the Department of Fair Trading in 1997.

Clearly, there is a role here for social workers in assisting local community groups to undertake this kind of project. Indeed, the student continued to assist the committee of founding members with its work and the group made several submissions for funding to the New South Wales Department of Housing, beginning in 1997. The group was successful in 1999 and received funding for nine dwellings for single people and families. Land was acquired to build five of the houses to the specifications of the cooperative and four existing local houses were bought.

The rental housing cooperative provides ongoing secure and affordable housing for a number of low-income families, single parents and single households, with many attendant advantages, including dignity and tenure, in a small rural town that otherwise has very limited available and affordable rental accommodation.

Reflective questions

- What kinds of skills and knowledge can social workers bring to the table to address housing shortages in regional, rural and remote settings?
- What kinds of skills and knowledge might the members of the housing cooperative have developed in the process of making the funding submission, purchasing the properties and being responsible for the long-term administration of a cooperative business?

CONCLUSION

Regional, rural and remote housing availability and affordability are impacted by the diversity of geography, recent housing changes like the resources boom, the sea- and tree-change phenomenon, rapid rises in housing prices and the slow and low level of wage rises in relation to accommodation costs. Currently, there is a housing affordability and availability crisis in Australia overall, with specific regional, rural and remote settlements being impacted in different ways. By using a contextual framework and solid policy analysis applied to specific places in regional, rural and remote settings, social workers can enable communities to develop human, financial and physical capital to address these housing shortages.

RECOMMENDED READING

Aged and Community Services Australia (2004) *Affordable Housing for Older People: A literature review.* Aged and Community Services Australia, Canberra, pp. 1–20.

Senate Select Committee on Housing Affordability (2008) *A Good House is Hard to Find: Housing affordability in Australia.* Commonwealth of Australia, Canberra.

5

DEVELOPING NEW APPROACHES TO MENTAL HEALTH IN FARM SETTINGS

Jane Maidment

CHAPTER OBJECTIVES

- To examine the unique pressures impacting upon the mental health of those engaged in agricultural and horticultural enterprise in rural Australia.
- To explore attitudes towards help-seeking among this particular population, together with ways of improving mental health literacy.
- To consider how social constructionist interpretations and a strengths-based approach to intervention might be used to guide practitioner responses to community mental health issues.
- To identify policy initiatives that have contributed to strengthening rural community responsiveness and the improvement of mental health status and literacy.

INTRODUCTION

The mental health status of farming communities in Australia has come into sharp focus in recent years. Multiple extreme weather events such as floods, droughts and bushfires, together with economic stringency due to declining terms of trade, have impacted upon the mental health and well-being of those living in rural communities. Within this context, rural practitioners need to be cognisant of how to respond effectively to mental distress among farming populations, and mindful about incorporating preventive capacity-building approaches into practice to support the resilience already present within most rural communities.

UNIQUE PRESSURES

Many rural communities in Australia do not have ready access to mental health services (Pierce et al., 2010). Together with a culture of stoicism and the continuing stigma associated with using mental health services, these circumstances create the conditions for mental illness to go unrecognised and untreated. In addition, declining numbers of people engaged in agricultural activity in Australia have resulted in a situation of growing physical and social isolation for those people who do farm (RIRDC & ACAHS, 2008). Key pressures identified by farmers themselves include a lack of finance, time, marketing and IT skills; difficulty in employing and retaining farm labour; increasing government regulation and compliance requirements; and the impact of severe weather events, with the cumulative effects of these conditions resulting in significant stress being brought to bear on family life and functioning (RIRDC & ACAHS, 2008: 7–8). Farming is clearly an environment in which multiple stressors are experienced, with research identifying that the strong association between 'maleness and farming' limits the capacity among farmers to acknowledge these pressures or seek help (Judd et al., 2006). Of central concern is the significantly higher rate of suicide among male farmers in Australia compared with that of non-farming rural men and the Australian male population more generally (Judd et al., 2006).

THE IMPACT OF WEATHER EVENTS AND NATURAL DISASTERS ON MENTAL HEALTH

Those living and working in rural and remote communities are radically dependent upon the environment to sustain their livelihoods. This is particularly so for people in the agricultural and horticultural sectors. Catastrophic weather events and natural disasters such as flooding and bushfires have an immediate and often devastating impact on personal and community well-being, as well as agricultural production. In recent years, long-term drought in many parts of Australia has impacted upon farm and horticultural income, necessitating engagement in off-farm employment, and resulting in prolonged financial worries and increased workloads for farming families. In some cases, severe drought has led to farming no longer being a viable option, with people having to sell stock and properties and find different forms of employment. The gravity of this type of loss is captured by Pugh and Cheers: 'losing a farm is not simply losing a job, it can mean leaving a way of life, losing a home and perhaps facing the end of a family tradition' (2010: 31).

Drought, severe flooding and fires often result in stock losses. Witnessing animals in distress and actively killing severely injured stock is emotionally taxing for farming people closely connected to the land. Experiencing a sense of loss and grief in these circumstances is normal, and has been identified as a 'business-related pressure' by farmers (RIRDC & ACAHS, 2008). The subsequent environmental degradation wrought by fires, floods and drought also prompts loss of hope and spirit, associated specifically with the destruction of the landscape. These ecological changes impact on the domains of personal well-being and sense of control (Sartore et al., 2008). In these circumstances, women in particular have registered a sense of spiritual loss associated with the destruction of the landscape. The ever-diminishing capacity to sustain a household garden is interpreted as the loss of a protective barrier between the home and an otherwise hostile environment (Sartore et al., 2008: 6).

Having no sense of control over climatic conditions, together with the need to make momentous lifestyle changes to survive financially, has placed rural-dwelling families and whole communities under significant strain (Tonna et al., 2009).

ATTITUDE TO HELP-SEEKING AND STIGMA

The defining discourse of rural Australia since the time of colonial settlement has been characterised by an attitude of silent stoicism, forbearance and individual struggle with the extreme nature of the country's environmental and geographical conditions. Within this context, maintaining an identity that privileges self-reliance, independence and resilience militates against help-seeking, particularly in matters relating to personal issues, emotional health and well-being. Lisa McColl (2007) illustrates this point in her research examining the links between bush identity and attitudes to mental health, which draws upon direct quotes from rural participants. One person observed that country people are proud people and because news can never be kept on a personal level (the whole community knows) then people don't want to be known to have mental health issues.

A second participant explained that:

people don't want to have the 'mental illness' title attached to them as it could mean a lack of business or respect within a small community. (McColl, 2007: 115)

These thoughts hint at the intertwined nature of business, personal and family life, where association with mental health troubles might well be perceived negatively, resulting in adverse social and economic outcomes. Dealing with problems alone is an entrenched culture—particularly for men—which regularly leads on to forms of drug and alcohol self-medication and substance abuse (Collins et al., 2009), in a milieu where there is often greater tolerance for heavy drinking (Pugh & Cheers, 2010).

While the general practitioner (GP) is regarded as the 'first port of call' for professional help in rural communities, participants in a number of studies identify people from informal networks such as family, friends and neighbours as being preferred sources of assistance (Collins et al., 2009). Since the advent of major health-promotion initiatives in Australia following drought and fire events, farmers have now begun to actively 'look out' for each other, especially in situations where particular problems are evident (Greenhill et al., 2009). These findings are supported by earlier research noting that 'despite the frequent bemoaning of the decline of community . . . durable and significant networks of kinship, belonging and association remain active in many places' (Crow & Allen, 1994, cited in Pugh & Cheers, 2010). At the same time, a closer examination of the nature of informal rural support systems suggests that conversations about farming difficulties are only acceptable within certain parameters, where issues are discussed in a positive solution-focused way without 'doom and gloom' (Judd et al., 2006: 6).

People living in small communities are reluctant to seek help through channels that identify themselves as providing mental health services. In particular, the shame, embarrassment and fear of stigma associated with experiencing mental health difficulties mean that many bush people—especially men—do not view accessing personal counselling as an acceptable way to address problems (McColl, 2007: 110).

While rural people report being unwilling to seek help for fear of being stigmatised, local responses will not necessarily be negative, and instead appear to be dependent upon the degree to which a person is considered to belong to the community in question (Barbopoulos & Clark, 2003, cited in Pugh & Cheers, 2010).

Together, these findings signal the importance of rural social work practitioners understanding the significance of 'place' and 'belonging' in a given community, where relationships are mediated via notions of kinship and neighbourhood networks, historical antecedents and occupation. With this understanding, practitioners can direct their energies towards strengthening existing informal support networks within rural communities, while establishing connections for those where few exist. In this regard, examining the notions associated with the social construction of rurality, coping and agriculture can assist practitioners to respond effectively.

Reluctance to engage with formal services means practitioners must find alternative avenues for providing health responses and increasing mental health literacy. Such measures would take account of the cultural norms and behaviours of those living in rural communities. One example of such an initiative is the 'Coach the Coach' program developed within rural Australian football clubs. Prompted by the deaths from suicide of a number of young men in a particular region, this initiative facilitates the training of football coaches to recognise signs of mental distress, while also facilitating the role of rural football clubs in becoming sites for early help-seeking (Pierce et al., 2010). Subtitled 'Don't wait, talk to a mate', the program targets key individuals with community credibility (such as coaches) to receive Mental Health First Aid (MHFA) training. These individuals then act as mentors, confidants and advocates within their clubs on matters relating to mental health. An evaluation of this program identified coaches' increased ability and confidence in recognising signs of mental distress and offering assistance. Participant coaches in the program also reported using the knowledge and skills developed through MHFA training in other settings, such as their workplace and home environments (Pierce et al., 2010), thus resulting in an increase in mental health literacy beyond the football club population.

Most importantly, the clubs have an existing organisational infrastructure to support such a project (Pierce et al., 2010), with those responsible for facilitating this initiative recognising football club culture as influential in shaping the social dynamics of rural communities. In this way, appreciating the nuanced flavour of the power dimensions that operate within rural communities enabled an effective mental health promotion strategy to be carried out. Engaging with a social constructionist perspective can therefore strengthen practitioner understanding of those living in different parts of rural Australia.

SOCIAL CONSTRUCTIONISM

A social constructionist approach to interpreting 'reality' privileges localised experiences, forms of knowledge and understanding (such as the influence of the football club in rural districts). In this regard, the way a given rural community is understood will be dependent upon local notions of social, political and economic influence, and this will be evidenced in prevailing dominant discourses. The ideas and beliefs that shape these discourses are created by expression of historically shared meanings that influence behaviour and language, and contribute to strongly held forms of community wisdom. Social relations between people and organisations are in turn mediated and negotiated through engagement with these discourses. From this perspective: 'The basic sense of a person's being emerges from and is an expression of his or her unique individual history within the dialogical context of the community of others and the physical world' (Greene & Kropf, 2009: 127). This way of understanding the world contrasts with a modernist perspective, where universal laws and theories, objective discovery and positivist paradigms are used to explain functioning.

As discussed in Chapter 1, particular discourses relating to rural and remote Australia have been promoted widely through the popular media, literature and agriculture industry. Images that speak to notions of hardy individualism, stoicism and resilience within a predominantly white, male-dominated culture prevail. This discourse privileges efforts to find solutions and be resourceful, and as such resonates well with adopting a strengths-based model for social work intervention.

RESILIENCE AND THE STRENGTHS PERSPECTIVE

While the dominant discourse of the bush militates against help-seeking endeavours, this ethos does promote a particular brand of resilience that is unique to rural communities. The nature of this resilience has been examined in some depth (Greenhill et al., 2009; Hegney et al., 2003), demonstrating that resilience is a protective factor in managing the stressors of rural living. Resilience within the context of rurality has been conceptualised as a process 'wherein an individual (e.g. farmer) displays positive adjustment such as psychological wellbeing or the absence of psychological distress despite experiencing adversity like severe drought' (Greenhill et al., 2009: 318). Identifying resilience as a *process* rather than a personality trait has implications for social work intervention. This particular research (Greenhill et al., 2009) identifies that resilience can be developed and promoted, prompting consideration of practice interventions that support this process. As such, using a *strengths-based* practice model is particularly relevant in a rural context, where clients already have a history of honouring strength and resilience, and are most likely to relate to a 'can do' philosophy.

In contrast to some earlier models of social work practice, which focus on personal deficits, diagnostic labelling and problem identification, the strengths-based approach is founded upon overt recognition of client and community resourcefulness. A strengths-based methodology incorporates the following principles:

- recognition that every individual, group, family and community has strengths
- an awareness that trauma, abuse, struggle and illness, while injurious, can also be sources of challenge and opportunity
- the concept that all people have the capacity to grow and change
- the belief that clients are the experts about their own lives, and
- recognition that every environment contains resources (Saleebey, 2002: 14–18).

This approach is underpinned by notions of healing and wholeness, as well as the generation of hope and empowerment. In order to assist with identification of client strengths, Clay Graybeal (2001) has developed the practical typology termed ROPES to guide work with clients. ROPES stands for ascertaining *Resources* (e.g. personal, family, organisational, community); creating *Options* (emphasis on choice: What can be accessed now? What is available and hasn't been tried?); creating *Possibilities* (e.g. future focus, imagination, creativity: What have you thought of trying but haven't tried yet?); identifying *Exceptions* (e.g. When is the problem not happening?

When is the problem different? How have you survived, endured, thrived?); and emphasising *Solutions* (focus on constructing solutions rather than solving problems: What's working now? What if a miracle happened? What would life then look like? What can you now do to create a piece of the miracle?) (Graybeal, 2001: 237). This typology provides a useful framework for direct client work in a rural setting.

While the dominant rural discourse calls attention to the experience of the white Australian male, to fully understand the milieu, the lived experiences of diverse groups including women, adolescents, older people and children in agricultural and horticultural farming communities need to be acknowledged. A recent Australian study of adolescents in a rural drought-affected area has demonstrated the cumulative effect on coping capacity of experiencing drought (Dean & Stain, 2010). Long-term exposure to drought is associated with an increase in emotional difficulties among adolescents. These difficulties related to family concerns, financial stress, worry about climate change and experience of an environment where death and loss were all too evident (Dean & Stain, 2010). Rural women do not rate their own health as positively as do their urban counterparts, with social factors having a considerable bearing on well-being (Harvey, 2009). The rural social context includes gendered expectations that women will be unpaid workers in the household, on the farm and through community volunteer efforts. These same women now need to engage in paid employment to further support family finances, creating a milieu of unmet expectations in a time-poor environment. Further, rural women historically have been service providers rather than service users (Coakes & Kelly, 1997, cited in Harvey, 2009: 355), so it has not been the norm to prevail upon professional 'helping' agencies.

CASE STUDY: DIRECT PRACTICE

Please read the scenario below, and in class groups record the role-plays according to the questions that follow:

Jim (66) and Karen (61) are married and have three children; two are adult and living independently, with one seventeen-year-old son, Mark, still living at home. For many years they have run a large cropping operation in the central-west grain belt of New South Wales. The property was originally farmed by Jim's parents, and Jim has spent his entire life on this piece of land. The area has experienced a prolonged period of drought and there have been three successive years of poor-quality crops, resulting in production of stock feed only. Karen has gained employment in the closest regional town, some 120 kilometres from the farm. She boards in town during the week and returns to the farm on weekends. One of their adult children lives interstate while the second (daughter Louise) has returned to the district after qualifying as a vet.

Due to the impact of the drought on production, the couple have had to steadily increase their mortgage to survive financially. For more than eighteen months, they have had ongoing conversations about 'selling up'. Jim is reluctant to do so and has become increasingly morose and irritable. Karen learns from a farming neighbour that Jim rarely leaves the house during the week, and has now taken to not answering the phone when she calls in the evening. According to the neighbour, Jim and Mark are arguing a fair bit. Louise visits her father and brother when she is out that way working, but with the vet practice to run and a young family, she does not have a lot of time to spend on the farm. Since the entire district is experiencing the drought, Louise has her own money worries, with farmers struggling to pay their vet bills.

You are a social worker based in a primary health practice in the regional town where Karen works. Karen calls you, saying she is worried about Jim and Mark, and asks if you could 'call in' to see them when you are next out that way. Karen tells you Jim is aware she is making contact with you. You phone Jim and he agrees that you can visit.

Reflections

- Role-play an in-depth face-to-face conversation with Jim where he talks about the farm, his family and his life. Use a strengths perspective to underpin your interviewing technique. The ROPES typology could be used to guide the interview process. This interview could take up to 30 minutes. (This is not your initial engagement conversation with Jim. At this stage you have a good rapport with

Jim and are now moving into the assessment/intervention stages of the social work process.) Video, audio record or have an observer watch this interview.

- After the interview, review the conversation you had with Jim and identify where you have used particular questioning techniques, reframing and solution-focused strategies. Note specifically where and how you might have approached the interview differently.
- From the way in which Jim describes his situation, decide what discourse he is using to make sense of his current reality.
- Next, role-play an in-depth face-to-face conversation you have with Mark at school where you ask him about the farm, his family, school and his social life. Use a strengths perspective to underpin your interviewing technique. Video, audio record or have an observer watching this interview, and debrief from this interview using the same process as with your role-play with Jim.
- Next, conduct telephone conversations (role-play in chairs back to back) with both Karen and Louise, assessing their views on the situation. Take particular note of how the telephone assessment and communication differ from face-to-face encounters.
- Identify some of the different 'life course' issues that Jim, Karen, Mark and Louise raise in their conversations with you (i.e. expectations about ageing, future planning, individual roles in the family, aspirations, obligations and responsibilities, and health).
- Go online and research some of the townships in the central-west grain belt of New South Wales. Look at their geography, industry, social, community and historical features. Identify factors that symbolise this region, examine the language and characterisation of agricultural activity associated with the area and read some of the tourist information. From your research, map out the overall discourse or key messages portrayed by the region. How might these 'messages' influence the way a practitioner engages with the community?

MENTAL HEALTH LITERACY AND POLICY RESPONSES

Some of the most significant rural health policy developments in recent years have related to improving mental health literacy among rural populations, in order to address issues of stigma, prevent suicide and promote general well-being. Several inquiries carried out in rural Australia identify lack of information, knowledge and awareness as contributing towards misconceptions about mental health status, with people still equating mental illness with a state of insanity (Collins et al., 2009; McColl, 2007).

Events such as the Drought Conference hosted by the Centre for Rural and Remote Health in 2003, and the Drought Summit organised by the New South Wales Farmers' Association in 2005 (RIRDC & ACAHS, 2008: 10) provided influential and informative public forums for education and discussion about the impacts of the prolonged drought on farmer mental health. Additional responses have emerged out of these events, including the creation of the Rural Mental Health Network, responsible for the development of the New South Wales Farmers' Blueprint for Maintaining the Mental Health and Wellbeing of People on New South Wales Farms (NSWFMHN, 2006). This blueprint identifies 23 areas for proactive attention, with the document currently being updated to address the broad range of issues impacting upon farming communities beyond the original focus on drought. Paradoxically, the severe flood events of 2010–11 have now affected many of the same regions in Queensland, New South Wales and Victoria previously impacted by drought, demonstrating the unpredictable and influential impact of weather conditions on farming as an enterprise.

Policy responses to address rural mental health literacy and capacity-building for service delivery have subsequently been implemented at both federal and state levels of government. These responses have included the Mental Health Services in Rural and Remote Areas Program, which began in 2006–07 with the establishment of a new standard measure for delivery of mental health services. This initiative has seen $60.4 million in federal funding being committed over five years to provide rural and remote areas with more allied and nursing mental health services. Rolled out in two stages, this particular program has focused on ensuring that service type and method of delivery are specifically designed for each rural and remote area, with funding targeted to identified geographical areas of need. More specifically, the 2007/08 federal budget followed up by announcing that a further $10.1 million would be made available to Divisions of General Practice to support mental health professionals and community leaders in responding to the impact of drought (Dunbar et al., 2007).

The most recent examples of federally funded service developments to address rural and remote mental health include upgrading the Royal Flying Doctor aircraft facilities and mental health support services for Far North Queensland (Australian Government, 2010b); and the provision of low-aromatic Opal fuel into Kakadu National Park to curb the effects of sustained petrol sniffing (Australian Government, 2010c).

Specific mental health policy initiatives at a state government level continue to be developed, with examples including the 2006 Drought Mental Health Assistance Package (DMHAP) delivered in New South Wales, which provided a comprehensive range of interventions to support both individuals in the community and those agencies delivering mental health services; the establishment in Victoria of a planning framework for public rural mental health services in 2007; the development of the Northern Territory Suicide Prevention Action Plan in 2009; and Western Australia's founding of the country's first Commission for Mental Health in 2010, with New South Wales soon to follow. Numerous other local responses have been trialled, including the 'Coach the Coach' program discussed earlier, which was developed in Victoria, with a similar initiative targeting Advisory and Extensions Agents for mental health first aid training to help support farmers in rural Queensland (Hossain et al., 2010).

Beyondblue is a bipartisan organisation funded by the state and territory governments with the specific mandate of raising community awareness about depression and anxiety. This agency has been particularly proactive in tackling the stigma associated with mental illness. In 2007, beyondblue launched 'Don't Beat About the Bush', a national campaign targeting rural drought-affected areas. The campaign used multiple strategies to encourage early identification of mental health symptoms, further developed accessible collaborative service delivery options, and focused on offering training to professionals and laypeople working in drought-stricken areas. Beyondblue's continued efforts to address mental health issues among farming people provide an avenue for resource networking and information dissemination about existing supports and services available in rural regions.

Online and telephone services have proved particularly helpful in providing information and responding to help-seeking among rural people. Examples of these services include the Centrelink Farmer Assistance Line, Bush Crisis Line and Support Services (for 24-hour support for rural health practitioners and their families), and the Rural Women's Telephone Counselling Service.

These initiatives appear to be having a positive impact on levels of mental health literacy among the rural population, with a recent investigation among South Australian farming families identifying good levels of mental health knowledge. In particular, farmers reported being proactive in their efforts to deal with physical, emotional and financial stressors and said they were mindful of looking out for each other (Greenhill et al., 2009).

IMPLICATIONS FOR RURAL SOCIAL WORK PRACTICE

A recent editorial in the *Australian Journal of Rural Health*, which focuses on mental health and well-being, signals potential strategies for rural social work practice (Allan, 2010). Julaine Allan notes that the best models for mental health service delivery in rural and remote regions are not always clear, and are often shaped more by opportunity than planning. The editorial makes the point that quality interventions need to include participation by informal networks and to take into account strengthening of social capital; that diverse local conditions and needs have to be accounted for, requiring flexibility in approaches to service delivery; and that better evidence of effectiveness and coordination of services is required (Allan, 2010: 3–4).

These observations demonstrate strong synergies between using community-development models of practice, targeting locally defined mental health priorities and focusing on capacity-building interventions. Such an approach requires practitioners to place less emphasis on traditional case-management models, instead adopting an approach where the idiosyncratic strengths of individual communities are drawn upon to create inventive service-delivery responses. This way of working requires the practitioner to have a very comprehensive and grounded knowledge of informal as well as formal community networks, an appreciation of the history of an area, and an understanding of the unique social norms associated with that history, including the dominant discourses, geographical place and emotional space occupied by the region. Such social work practice calls for a holistic understanding of community beyond individual interventions, where the formal and informal power dimensions operating at all levels of the social strata are well understood and constructively mobilised to strengthen mental health responses.

The call made by Allan (2010) to strengthen rural mental health interventions through robust evaluation also signals some clear priorities for social work as a discipline. Currently, extremely low levels of knowledge and confidence in conducting research and evaluation have been identified among social work practitioners (Beddoe, 2010), pointing to the urgent need for practitioners to engage in further learning to address this practice imperative and gap in the professional knowledge. In order for practitioners to argue for the pursuit of localised community-embedded responses to mental health issues, the efficacy of these initiatives will need to be proven. The call for development of practitioner research knowledge and confidence is not an issue solely confined to those working in rural communities. Accessible advanced professional development opportunities to learn about undertaking practice research could potentially be provided online, in order for social workers in rural, regional and urban areas to develop these skills together.

Despite many rural areas still experiencing difficulties in accessing mental health services, increased attention, funding and service development in the area of mental health are evident across rural Australia. Appreciation of the importance of mental health is now definitely 'on the agenda' in rural communities. Awareness-raising initiatives regarding mental health status could potentially be reshaping former dominant social norms that called for hard-core stoicism and silent forbearance among farming populations. The inherent dangers of these particular belief systems have been challenged by increasing mental health literacy within the farming sector. Policy and practice interventions appear to work best when they have emerged out of, and are shaped by, the unique social norms present in specific rural communities. Social work practitioners therefore must become as one with the community and its needs, to accurately tap into actual and potential resources for intervention, and to gain a sense of the best way to foster community well-being. This approach requires a combination of the art and science of social work practice, where the subjective experiences of individuals and groups living in particular rural communities are responded to in ways that may be quite unique, yet still subject to critical appraisal and robust evaluation processes.

RECOMMENDED READING

Graybeal, C. (2001), Strengths-based social work assessment: Transforming the dominant paradigm. *Families in Society: Journal of Contemporary Human Services*, 82(3), 233–43.

McColl, L. (2007) The influence of bush identity on attitudes to mental health in a Queensland community. *Rural Society*, 17(2), 107–24.

Pierce, D., Liaw, S.T., Dobell, J. & Anderson, R. (2010) Australian football club leaders as mental health advocates: An investigation of the Coach the Coach project. *International Journal of Mental Health Systems*, 4, 10.

6

EMPLOYING AND SUPPORTING YOUNG PEOPLE'S BELONGING IN RURAL TOWNS

Lesley Chenoweth

CHAPTER OBJECTIVES

- To investigate the impact of population shifts on rural livelihoods.
- To explore the issues associated with employment for rural young people.
- To outline the relevant policy and practice contexts and implications.

INTRODUCTION

For most young people in Australia, decisions about their future work and career are rich with possibilities and choices. Higher education has become a pathway for increasing numbers of Australian school leavers over recent years. Vocation education options have proliferated, often in ever-changing fields and industries, and employment prospects in many states are healthy. However, most of these choices—especially for further education—are available mainly in urban or larger centres. For young people in rural areas, choices are fewer for those wishing to remain in their communities. Employment for rural young people can pose certain challenges not only for them and their families but also for their communities. Some of the most innovative examples of how these issues can be tackled are to be found in rural communities and settlements. These examples give us rich insights into community resilience and creativity when it comes to solving seemingly intractable problems.

The picture of rural Australia has transformed over recent years in such a way that the significant message about contemporary rural communities now reflects diversity and change. On one hand, the populations of many inland centres have been declining for decades, and for many small rural communities the experience has been of reduced services and infrastructure, a dwindling agricultural base and financial hardship (Eacott & Sonn, 2006). On the other hand, many regional centres have grown and prospered as mining interests have created jobs in infrastructure and commerce. The populations of some rural towns have grown in response to the demand for commerce and services by the mining and agricultural industries. However, for some young people growing up in rural communities, the lack of choice has created uncertainty. Many choose to leave their families and communities to seek a future in urban and larger regional centres. Others, with few local job prospects, experience poverty and personal difficulties.

The shifts and changes in the population have brought concomitant differences in rates of employment and workforce patterns. Trends such as the casualisation of the agricultural labour force, the fly-in/fly-out model of employment in mining areas, and the increase in migration of sea- and tree-changers to smaller communities have created different patterns of livelihood for rural dwellers.

These changes have considerable implications for rural social work practice. Responding to the employment needs of young people in rural communities requires approaches that are community based and tied in with economic development initiatives. Social workers therefore need a working knowledge of policy responses across a number of areas of government. Programs specifically created to address social problems such as the impact of drought, economic uncertainty and unemployment, and the effect of those events and circumstances on mental health, will offer points for leverage and change. In the main, community-development approaches will be most apt for working in communities undergoing change.

This chapter outlines the locational context and central issues around employment for young people in rural communities. It focuses on the population gaps and trends that have occurred in rural communities, and discusses the consequent labour force and employment issues. The chapter explores service delivery models and underlying theory—particularly the contributions of rural sociology and theories of space and place. The driving policy frameworks of strengthening communities and building social capital are also analysed. Finally, the chapter evaluates the key methods for practice adopted in this field, and illustrates these with an example of community capacity-building. The chapter focuses particularly on the impacts of the shift of young people away from rural settlements and what this has meant for the livelihoods of rural communities.

THE CONTEXT OF RURAL AUSTRALIA

Rural Australia comprises many diverse and dynamic environments. These include the complexity of natural, economic and social environments and the myriad of interrelationships they engender. Small communities face a range of challenges. For many inland and remote communities, land-use degradation, long droughts, sudden floods, climate change and the dominant issue of water have gained prominent attention and aroused concern. Economic results from this have included a decline in agriculture and farming and the loss of key services to many rural centres. Reduced government and private services in small rural towns have further contributed to the loss of employment opportunities. Many coastal communities have experienced population growth above the national average as sea-changers moved from capital cities to smaller centres. Anne M. Garnett and Philip Lewis (2007) observe that population changes are not mirrored by employment changes.

Coastal communities have attracted people, but largely for reasons of amenity and social factors rather than jobs. A particular impact of these factors has been the dramatic loss of young people from rural areas, as they are forced to move to larger cities in search of higher education and employment opportunities (Forth, 2001; Rogers & Ryan, 2001). These economic impacts have brought about changes in the social fabric of many rural communities, including a higher proportion of ageing people, ill-health, poverty and unemployment (Alston, 2004a).

RURAL LIVELIHOODS

The traditional view of Australian rural livelihoods has been one strongly based in farming and agricultural production. The family farm can still be regarded as a pillar of rural industry; however, as indicated in Chapter 1, there has been a significant shift to global multinational agricultural enterprises (Macadam et al., 2004).

Robyn Eversole (2004) argues that the shift towards corporate farming and national/international retail chains providing local goods and services has meant a move away from local ownership. Hence there is a widening gap between local goals and aspirations, and the sources of economic prosperity. This translates into a situation where many rural enterprises are producing wealth for a distant owner, but at the cost of simultaneously eroding the social fabric and networks in local communities.

Large-scale crops and grazing enterprises rely more on an itinerant workforce or seasonal employment than on a permanent rural workforce employed within family agricultural concerns. The pattern of contract labour and seasonal activities has created a rural job market that is characterised by unskilled, low-paid and intermittent employment. The lack of skills, coupled with financial hardship and distance, creates barriers to rural young people finding out about opportunities, gaining higher education, and acquiring better paid jobs and more skills (Kilpatrick & Abbott-Chapman, 2002).

A number of pressing economic and social issues emerge for residents of such communities, issues which are heightened for young people seeking a future, a career and further education.

CENTRAL ISSUES

Against these contextual social and demographic factors, it is not surprising that the career and lifestyle choices of rural young people have raised concerns. Rural youth are described as disadvantaged economically, educationally and socially (Alston, 2004a; Morgan, 2007). For example, faced with fewer educational facilities close to home, they tend to leave school earlier than their urban counterparts, consequently becoming even less competitive in the job market (Alloway & Dalley-Trim, 2009). Many rural communities are facing shrinking employment opportunities and juggling economic decline. Young people are therefore far less likely to obtain part-time work while still at school, to shore up some degree of financial independence to carry through to higher education afterwards. Families, too, are less likely to be in a position to offer financial support for housing, transport and study expenses for the move to a larger centre with greater educational opportunities.

Faced with uncertain employment and financial futures, the psychological and social impacts on young people are exacerbated. Mental health issues, drug and alcohol use are increased for this population. However, rural young people also have less access to the counselling, drug and alcohol and personal support services that they are more likely to need (Morgan, 2007).

Several factors influencing young people's decisions to stay or move from their rural community have been identified in the research literature. Aspirations of young people in rural communities are generally similar to those of all young people—that is, they want to be something (Alloway & Dalley-Trim, 2009). However, a combination of economic, social and personal issues affects these aspirations.

The major disincentive to moving away is financial, as the cost of living away from home is prohibitive for many young people and their families (Alloway & Dalley-Trim, 2009). Many families have suffered significant financial losses, and therefore are no longer in a position to support their young person to move away to study or work. However, some metropolitan universities offering rural and remote scholarships assist some of these young people in paying rental costs. Some young people, due to their family's low income, also gain access to government payments that contribute to paying for living costs in the city. Often a cohort of young people will leave a town at a similar time and support each other by sharing short-term accommodation in the city.

Attachment to place and level of satisfaction with community are other key factors that drive some young people to move away and keep others close to home. Many young people identify the benefits of a rural lifestyle and attachment to home and family as something which they want to hold onto—or at least return to after completing their education. As Kim Kirstein and Suniti Bandranaike (2004) point out from their study of young people in Richmond, Queensland:

> growing up in a small, close-knit community provides a sense of safety, unlimited freedom, and opportunities to drive cars, ride motor bikes and horses, and go swimming in rivers. As a result of these childhood experiences some Richmond youth also expressed a desire to return to Richmond to raise a family or after completing their studies and gaining work experience.

This study highlighted the dilemma that some young people in the study encountered, and of which they were acutely aware. They wanted to remain at home enjoying the country lifestyle and in close contact with family, yet realised that gaining a good education was not an option in Richmond. As one of the participants commented about being sent to boarding school:

> 'a necessary evil' I guess you could call it. You prefer to be home but you know you gotta be there. It wasn't that bad, you couldn't do what you want, you could only go into town for two hours once a week. (Richmond Youth Living in Townsville 7, pers. comm., 25 February 2004)

Non-completion of high school education is one of the most pressing issues for rural young people (Morgan, 2007). The flow-on effect of this is an increased risk of unemployment, or under-employment in low-skilled areas with unstable job opportunities.

POLICY CONTEXT

General economic and social policies, as well as more targeted rural regional policy, contribute to the complex interplay of initiatives, programs, funding and service provision impacting upon the lived experience and aspirations of Australia's young rural citizens. In considering the policy landscape faced by these young Australians, it is necessary to take into consideration broad policy directions, targeted policy initiatives and the impact of microeconomic reform.

Philip Morgan (2007) comprehensively summarises the key broad policy agendas around education, employment and welfare. While the intent of these national policies is to provide the necessary education, training and employment options for all young people, these options have not been readily accessible to rural young people, and there has been little support offered to assist them to navigate these confusing agendas and experiences. However, schools and social workers can play a major role in assisting students to understand these policies and to facilitate their navigation of the policy implications for their day-to-day lives.

What policy frameworks are relevant to rural communities, and in particular young people, to address these issues? First, it is important to confront the reality that regional development encompasses a number of different policy areas, including infrastructure, finance, environment and social policy. Because of this cross-disciplinarity, defining regional development is a slippery concept. Regional development is perhaps best viewed as 'a holistic process whereby the environmental, economic, social and cultural resources of a region are harnessed for sustainable progress in ways that reflect the comparative advantages offered by a particular geographic area' (Australian Local Government Association, www.alga.asn.au).

For social work practitioners entering this field, several key policy areas might be canvassed. A number of questions arise within each policy domain. When you have read this chapter, return to this section and consider these questions:

- *Economic and business development.* How can rural enterprises be created, supported and developed? What opportunities exist for working with communities around business development?
- *Educational policy and programs.* What initiatives are available that are aimed at improving access to education, vocational training and university? Do these initiatives provide financial incentives, local access points and a focus on learning communities?
- *Health and mental health policies.* What policy initiatives specifically offer programs and resources for rural young people living with mental illness, such as depression?
- *Community capacity-building that focuses on human and social capital development.* How can young people be included in the development of social capital and contribute to the general community?
- *Welfare benefits and reform.* What are the impacts of changes to welfare policies for rural young people? Are rural youth disadvantaged by changes to welfare eligibility?

Such questions need to inform a social work practice approach when working with rural youth around employment and their future goals. It is through exploration and analysis of these policies that practitioners can be better informed to assist individuals and communities to access relevant programs and services, to navigate the policy maze and to lobby for resources that are needed but not readily available.

THEORY AND METHOD FOR COMMUNITY DEVELOPMENT

On reviewing the policy and program context for this practice area, it quickly becomes apparent that this is an issue that spans individual, family and community issues, involves a range of service systems and is a whole-of-community concern. Like much rural practice, working on these issues with rural young people and their employment indicates community development as a preferable approach. Moreover, policies that have community-building as their goal are likely to provide the best framework for practice. Theories that best inform rural community development practice are varied; however, two key bodies of theory provide a constructive starting point for practice: theories of social capital and theories of place. Social capital theories provide useful frames for understanding community networks and, more importantly, how community capacity can be developed and grown. Social capital has been described as the 'raw material' of society, created as it is from the array of everyday interactions between people, and as the social fabric or glue that makes us human. At a more practical level, social capital refers to the networks and norms that allow people to work together to resolve problems and achieve common goals. This allows for consideration of the relationship between social and economic factors in communities.

The second theoretical platform for practice focuses on the notion of place and people's relationship to it. People and places are connected in complex ways, and in rural communities this relationship appears to be contested. Place is inextricably linked to the social, and is constantly being negotiated across social, cultural, historical and physical aspects of the environment. In rural areas, the history of and cultural meanings attached to landscape are influenced by the constant changing of place through natural events such as floods, droughts and different land uses. Kerry-Elizabeth Allen (2002) argues that people desire to belong somewhere, either in a place or in space within that place, and that it is within that space that social relations are constructed. It is crucial to point out here that 'rural' is not one homogeneous space, but rather a multiplicity of spaces in which social relations are negotiated and meanings are constructed. For young people in rural areas, different social spaces exist around family, community, farm, peers and landscape. An understanding of how the dimensions of all these places shape human experience not only helps us analyse the situation but also offers ways of thinking about solutions to problems. It also provides a useful safeguard to thinking about what might not work—for example, is the attachment to place so strong that even the economic advantage of moving to a larger centre cannot provide sufficient impetus to leave, and indeed, would doing so have serious emotional consequences?

Over the past two decades, community development—especially in rural areas—has become focused on the notion of 'capacity-building'.

There has been a growing interest in developing the ability of local communities, groups and networks to contribute to social and economic development. At a policy level, this has become enshrined in the idea of the triple bottom line—that is, that economic, social and environmental issues are equally important and inextricably linked. Strengthening people's capacity to determine values and priorities across all of these domains and to initiate actions to address their concerns has become the basis for much community development. It could be argued that this approach is a 'band-aid' solution, focusing attention on local community problems or deficits rather than much wider structural social issues, such as unemployment or social exclusion. It also relies heavily on volunteers and voluntary efforts when the real need is for more health and social services in rural communities.

Deborah Eade (1997) argues that practice in this context is not merely a set of predetermined interventions, but rather an overall approach that incorporates the following principles:

- Capacity-building must not be seen in isolation.
- All community members have capacities that may not be obvious, and it may take time to discover them.
- To be inclusive, interventions must take into account different and sometimes negative ways in which the impacts will be experienced.
- Flexibility is important, but this must not be at the expense of a loss of direction with regard to wider processes of social and economic transformation.
- Capacity-building is not 'doing development' on the cheap or against the clock.
- Capacity-building is not risk-free.

CASE STUDY: THE GROOVE CAFE

Channeltown is a rural centre with a population of approximately 19 000 located in a non-metropolitan zone some 350 kilometres from the state capital. Largely reliant on agriculture, the town has had its share of economic blows from lower commodity prices, drought and the closure of several key services in recent years. A number of businesses have closed since the economic downturn and job opportunities are few and seasonal. There has been a move to establish some rural tourism in the area and early indicators look promising, though this is in its infancy. Channeltown High School has approximately 800 students from the town and surrounding areas. Most students leave at or before Year 10.

In response to increasing numbers of young people leaving school with no job prospects, and more young people reluctantly opting to leave the town to look for work in larger centres, the Channeltown Social Issues Committee held a series of community consultations and specifically included young people. There were real concerns after a young man aged seventeen committed suicide after failing to find work when he left school at sixteen.

These consultations revealed that Channeltown's young citizens faced a number of challenges, and felt they were under increasing pressure to secure some sort of future for themselves. Small-group meetings were held with young people, with the goal of determining what they needed to feel part of the community. Young people indicated that they wanted a space of their own to hang out, access to the internet, and to get help and advice on a range of problems they did not want to discuss with family members or others.

This process of consultation and developing of recommendations led to the establishment of the Channeltown Youth Action Committee (CYAC), made up of young people and some stakeholders from local business, government and community organisations. Ultimately, the Groove Cafe was established. The cafe began in premises in the main street provided free of charge by the local council. Initially operating as a part-time drop-in centre for local young people, and run by volunteers—largely young people themselves—the cafe evolved over time into a one-stop shop for several services. The CYAC worked with local council personnel to apply for a seeding grant to develop facilities in the cafe. It was through this that the CYAC was able to employ a part-time community worker, Seth, who had worked in other rural areas as a youth worker and had some experience of issues around unemployment in larger centres.

Seth brought new skills and knowledge to CYAC and the cafe. He worked closely with the young people and the broader community to establish key areas of need. Attracting further one-off grants and raising funds through operating as a small part-time internet cafe, Groove Cafe slowly developed other services and activities over the next three years. These included:

- a space for young people that became an access point for other services
- a venue for vocational training and assistance in developing job applications
- an access point for advertising local job vacancies
- a small business in the town that employed young people and trained them in hospitality
- a functioning focus point for partnerships between young people and local businesses, and
- a more positive image of young people within the broader community.

The cafe has not been without its challenges, and young people in Channeltown still experience many difficulties. CYAC identified needs for counselling services, for increased training and employment opportunities for young people who wished to stay in Channeltown, and for more housing and accommodation options for young people. Groove Cafe has provided a stronger sense of belonging for many young people, a space of their own, while also contributing to building the capacity of the community in a range of ways.

Reflective questions

- Consider the relationship between education and sustainable rural communities. What are the key factors affecting this relationship? What strategies might be adopted to increase the participation in higher education of young rural Australians? How effective do you think these strategies might be and how would you determine their effectiveness?
- Imagine you are the community development worker employed to set up the Groove Cafe. What key issues would you need to consider in embarking on this project? How would you engage all the relevant people? Would your approach differ if you were a local? Someone from outside? If so, how?

CASE STUDY: CAPACITY-BUILDING IN REDROO

Redroo is a remote town of 7000 people situated 200 kilometres from the provincial centre of Emu Siding (population
23 000). Redroo's economy has largely been based on grazing
and providing services to surrounding properties, and it is
the closest service centre to a number of Indigenous communities in the area. There is minor tourism based on fishing
and hunting during the season. Redroo was also chosen as
one of eight statewide locations for a new state government
Community Capacity Project. Under this project, a community
worker was employed to work with the community to address
the issues it identified as important. These workers also had
links into government at all levels. Flo, a community worker
originally from a nearby town with several years' rural experience, was appointed to this position. One of the key issues
the community identified concerned the future for the town's
young people. Many dropped out of school and were therefore
under-skilled. There were too few local jobs for young people
in the town, and even those that did exist were usually not
offered to young people by industry.

Over a series of public meetings and gatherings, the community worked on forging partnerships between schools, post-
secondary institutions, local businesses and parents. A group
of six people, representing parents, young people, industry, the
health and social sector, schools, post-secondary and government, was charged with the task of getting to the bottom of
the issues and coming up with some solutions. These were
then brought back to the wider group. Flo was to facilitate this
process over a two-day workshop with the six representatives.
They grappled with the main issues, different opinions and
problems. Using group facilitation skills to ensure that every
participant had ample opportunity for frank and open sharing
of ideas, Flo still had to keep the group focused on solutions
by bringing the group back to the main task—strategy. In these
situations, having a skilled facilitator is key and the group
agreed on the following issues:

- Parents and schools needed to work together to keep young
  people in school and provide options for those leaving.
  Ideas here included part-time school and part-time work

experience or training. It was also acknowledged that some young people did not complete school and they should not be labelled as failures because of this.

- There was a need to build career aspirations. Schools needed to start career planning earlier (e.g. Years 2–3), with a focus on building a work ethic and aspirations. Students needed better labour market information about jobs coming up in the next decade and the requisite skills and qualifications to perform them.
- Industry needed to provide better information and more training on the job for youth and better policies related to job performance. Industry standards were very rigid, so youth were either not hired or were fired quickly. The group saw the need for a shift to 'keeping young people employed rather than kicking them out'.
- Post-secondary training was needed to deliver 'closer to home' opportunities and educational offerings needed to change so they were less focused on 'come-to-us' and 'traditional' trades. Easier entrance to post-secondary training and more 'Jack/Jill of all trades' offerings were needed— for example, basic skills such as workplace safety, and how to use and care for tools, which applied to many jobs.

A few months after the community began this process, a new mining operation, Outback Metals Australia (OMA), announced that it was going to open outside of Redroo. This was a smaller company which had operated on the fly-in/fly-out workforce model in its previous ventures. This offered few local benefits, limited jobs to untrained locals and even fewer to youth.

The community saw this as its lucky break—it had already done the preliminary work and here was an opportunity to put its ideas into practice. Drawing on Flo's networks, community representatives met with the relevant government departments for advice and support. They started a process to work out a partnership with OMA. For once, this was to be on the community's terms and not imposed on them. They held many meetings and workshops involving an expanded network. They invited industry and mine representatives into this process.

Elements of this partnership included:

- The schools developed career option programs related to the mine, which linked into post-secondary training for the sector.
- The government subsidised some of the jobs created at the mine to allow for training on the job for local people—an obvious financial incentive to the company and a vital link to the partnership.
- The community invited the company to be a community partner in sports and cultural events. This was to invite the company to be part of the community, not just donating money or goods—a process again supported and facilitated through Flo.
- Businesses struck a deal to supply some local products to the mine (catering, building supplies, some trucking services). This allowed an increase in business and some young people were trained to manage small service businesses. Government programs for small business were accessed to support these micro-enterprises.

In reflecting on this whole process, the community worked with Flo to draw out some of the key learning over the years. The insights gained provide an instructive summary for any beginning rural community practitioner. First, past approaches do not always work in the current context. Conditions require a holistic process that involves everyone, and this needs to be proactive. Leaving it to parents and schools or industry and an open labour market alone cannot address these issues. Communities also need to think beyond the immediate. Industry is short term and cannot provide jobs forever. More current labour market information is needed, especially ways to use it into the next ten to 25 years. This includes information about what kind of jobs will be required and what training is needed.

Communities have more power than they often realise— they can insist on hiring and buying locally. Government is also a key player and can give more than support. It can make or break industry deals. Similarly, communities really need to buy in and be involved in new ways.

A second set of insights arose concerning the importance of community workers when it comes to achieving community goals. Their skills are needed to help the process. Community workers can provide consistency and need to remain in place. Flo worked with this community on partnership-building for almost three years. Sustainable outcomes need longer time-frames.

Finally, culture and belonging in communities includes industry and government, not just local people and their friends. The people who come and go are part of the community too.

Reflective questions

- The Redroo process continued over several years, with one community worker staying the distance. What do you think would have happened if Flo had left after a year? Would the Redroo group have continued? If so, in what ways?
- The central goal in this example was capacity-building. How was capacity developed? Whose capacity? Were any sectors of the community disadvantaged by this partnership-building? Who were they, and in what ways were they disadvantaged?
- A major feature of the Redroo process was the relationships between government and the local community. Indeed, an element of its success was the contribution of incentives and specific support programs by government. But to do this there needs to be a foundation of trust. How do you think tensions between local and central government could be resolved, and how can trust be developed? What is the role of the social worker in this?

CONCLUSION

This chapter has examined the transition from school to work or higher education for young people living in rural communities. The impact on young rural people's employment of population shifts, changing industry profiles and unavailability of post-school education and training has been significant. The assumption that all young people opt to leave for larger centres denies the importance of belonging, and attachment to place and family for young people. Such migrations also contribute to the decline in rural livelihoods and communities. For practitioners working in such contexts, community-building frameworks and community-development approaches have much to offer, especially where new industry initiatives are occurring. As the examples in this chapter have illustrated, employment options can be created when whole communities come together with skilled workers to collaborate towards a common purpose.

RECOMMENDED READING

Alloway, N. & Dalley-Trim, L. (2009) High and dry in rural Australia: Obstacles to student aspirations and achievements. *Rural Society*, 19(1), 49–59.

Australian Local Government Association, <www.alga.asn.au>.

Eacott, C. & Sonn, C. (2006) Exploring youth experiences of their communities: Place attachment and reasons for migration. *Rural Society*, 16(2), 199–214.

7

CAREGIVING IN SMALL RURAL AND REGIONAL TOWNS

Wendy Bowles

CHAPTER OBJECTIVES

- To introduce the disability field of practice for social workers within the context of small towns in Australia.
- To introduce the broader international and national theoretical and policy context within which disability services operate.
- To identify key features of disability practice for social workers in rural Australia, including advantages, opportunities and challenges.

INTRODUCTION

It was our family's move to a small regional community that gave me the opportunity to achieve what I have in my life so far. The acceptance and encouragement I found in that community, in contrast to the exclusion I experienced in the city, is the reason I celebrate International Day for People with a Disability as a day to celebrate small communities and what they can do for the people who live there.

—Jessica Smith, Paralympian and invited speaker for International Day for People with a Disability, West Wyalong, New South Wales, 3 December 2010

This chapter introduces social work with people with disabilities in small towns in Australia. Many of the examples are drawn from West Wyalong, a small town of around 3000 people in south-western

New South Wales (Bland Shire Council, 2011) and the site for Jessica Smith's speech to mark International Day for People with a Disability 2010, quoted above.

THE CONTEXT OF DISABILITY, SMALL TOWNS AND REGIONAL AND REMOTE LIFE

In order to work effectively with people with disabilities, their families and networks in small towns, contextual issues have to be understood and taken into account. This means engaging with paradox. On one hand, research evidence demonstrates serious levels of disadvantage. The Australian Institute of Health and Welfare (AIHW) singles out Indigenous people, rural people and people with disabilities as three of the most disadvantaged population groups within the general Australian population (Bullock, 2010). How is it, then, that Jessica Smith, the Paralympian quoted at the beginning of this chapter, speaks so highly of life in a small Australian town—especially as she was initially raised in the city, where services for people with disabilities are so much more readily available (Smith, 2010)? Even the AIHW, in the midst of describing the disadvantage experienced by rural and regional Australians, comments on the 'unique and enjoyable lifestyle' savoured by so many people in rural areas, and goes on to highlight that personal safety, community connection and general well-being are higher in some rural areas than in urban areas (Bullock, 2010: 246). Clearly there are also positives to living and working in small towns, and regional and rural areas. This chapter attempts to explore some aspects of this contradictory situation for social workers in the disability field.

Research shows that services for people with disabilities and their supporters tend to be scarce in small towns, and in rural and regional areas, in comparison to urban areas. In the late 1990s, Lindsay Gething (1997) documented the 'double disadvantage' faced by people with a disability and their carers in rural and remote New South Wales. She noted the lack of access to specialist services, difficulties with transport, and the long distances families had to travel to visit specialists in the city, as well as the isolation experienced by families living with a member with a disability. She also highlighted the acute lack of respite services, protection of rights, disability awareness education, housing, employment, education, access to information, and availability of aids and equipment for rural people with disabilities and their supporters.

Since Gething's paper, several studies into specific disability issues have documented the barriers preventing equitable access to services for rural people with disabilities. These include studies of rural people with developmental disabilities (Iacono et al., 2003), mental health issues (Murray et al., 2004), traumatic head injuries (Kingston et al., 2010), acquired brain injury (Parsons & Stanley, 2008) and spinal cord injury (Youngt et al., 2004). The recent report *Shut Out: The Experience of People with Disabilities: National Disability Strategy Consultation Report* (National People with Disabilities and Carers Council, 2009) demonstrates that little has changed for people with disabilities in the twelve years since Gething's work was published.

One critical issue for the context of the disability field in small towns is the situation faced by Aboriginal and Torres Strait Islander peoples. The AIHW makes the point that Indigenous people's rates of disadvantage are even more severe than those of rural and regional communities generally (Bullock, 2010: 246). Indigenous Australians have a lower quality of life, die much younger and experience poorer health and higher levels of disability than their non-Indigenous counterparts (Bullock, 2010: 228). The difference of ten to twelve years in life expectancy between Indigenous and non-Indigenous Australians is the widest health gap between indigenous and non-indigenous populations internationally, and the only one that is increasing (Zhao et al., 2010).

One of the main reasons for this gap is the significant levels of socio-economic disadvantage suffered by Indigenous peoples (Bullock, 2010: 229). The Council of Australian Governments (COAG) recognised this shameful state of affairs in November 2008 when it committed to six specific targets to improve aspects of life for Indigenous peoples in its *Closing the Gap* agreement. These included targets in health, mortality rates, education and employment (Australian Government, 2010a). The *Closing the Gap* strategy, in itself, demonstrates the multi-dimensional nature of the problems confronting Aboriginal and Torres Strait Islander peoples in Australia.

A single summary measure that takes into account both death and illness is 'disability-adjusted life years' (DALY), which is the sum of years of life lost due to premature death, and healthy years of life lost due to disability. On this measure, the AIHW estimates that two-thirds of the Indigenous health gap is due to mortality, and one-third due to disability. The AIHW estimates that after age differences are taken into account, Indigenous Australians experience around twice the rate of disability faced by non-Indigenous Australians (Bullock, 2010: 233). There is evidence that this gap is getting worse: Yuejen Zhao and colleagues' (2010) analysis of DALY scores between Indigenous and non-Indigenous groups in the Northern Territory shows that the gap is widening, with Indigenous people in the Northern Territory living longer, with increasing levels of disability and disease, compared with the non-Indigenous population, whose DALY scores remain static.

Compounding this larger burden of disability for Aboriginal and Torres Strait Islander peoples is their much lower use of services compared with the general population. Research reports from around Australia document how Aboriginal and Torres Strait Islander people are excluded from disability services, largely due to services being culturally unsafe or insensitive. These reports exhort disability services to improve their accessibility for and engagement with Indigenous Australians (Disability Services Commission, 2006; NSW Ombudsman, 2010). In New South Wales, the ADHC reports that Aboriginal and Torres Strait Islander peoples are more likely to provide support to people with disabilities than the rest of the population, noting that '12.4 per cent of Aboriginal people were providing assistance [to people with disabilities] compared to 10.4 per cent of the general population' (NSW Department of Human Services, 2009: 4).

CENTRAL ISSUES FOR PROFESSIONALS

While there is a growing amount of literature about rural and regional health and welfare workers in Australia, so far there is comparatively little research available about rural and regional disability workers. Therefore, some of the discussion in this chapter relies on the personal experience and observations of the author.

Due to the dwindling populations, services and consequently numbers of health and welfare professionals in small towns, pressures on these personnel are greater now than they were in the past. Studies into a range of health and welfare staff (AIHW, 2009b), and social workers specifically (Cheers et al., 2007), reveal growing professional isolation, shrinking opportunities for professional development and supervision, longer hours of work and the tendency to be on call more often, or to be called out of hours because the worker's personal address is known.

While on one hand professionals in small towns may well be the sole representative of their discipline, on the other they tend to work closely with colleagues from different disciplines. In addition to building local support networks with a range of disciplines, professionals sometimes overcome professional isolation by establishing rural interest groups within their discipline, travelling long distances to meet for conferences, and using video and teleconference links for meetings. The Victorian Rural Social Work Action Group (Mason, 2009) is a good example of such a group. Social workers may also develop supervision and peer-support relationships with colleagues at a distance, substituting face-to-face meetings with teleconferences or more sophisticated electronic communication, depending on its availability.

Along with other rural and regional workers, social workers working with people with disabilities and their families in small towns learn to work within the context of their local community, and to deal with the interdependencies, multiple relationships and complex role boundary negotiations that take place as a result (Gregory et al., 2007). This means a different type of client–worker relationship than the more anonymous professional relationship assumed by urban-based workers.

Instead of beginning their relationship with a referral or request for service, as would happen in the city, in small towns it is likely that the worker and the client will know quite a bit about each other before they work together. This includes information about family history and relationships as well as possibly belonging to the same local organisations. Under normal circumstances these shared relationships are a valued part of small communities' social capital and are the very links through which local people support each other in times of need (Onyx et al., 2007). In the initial phases of their working relationship both client and worker might need to reassess whether what they 'know' about the other is accurate. Whereas in larger regional centres social workers might negotiate with clients about whether or not to greet each other in public, this is not usually an issue in small communities, where people tend to greet each other as a matter of courtesy.

Paradoxically, in small communities where so much personal information is public, privacy can be guarded fiercely. There is also a strong culture of self-reliance and people solving their own problems. Those needing assistance with personal issues may seek professional services outside their local communities to ensure confidentiality. Locally, any professional with a reputation for gossiping will be shunned.

In the right environment, such transparency can lead to more honest and respectful interactions on both sides; there is a 'down-to-earth' quality to professional relationships between people who interact with each other across different roles in a small community. John Scascighini, a radiographer living and working in West Wyalong, sums up some of the boundary issues for professionals in small communities:

> I knew a high percentage of my patients by their first name. I played sport with them, they were guests in my home, my kids went to school with their kids. This can be good but it also presents difficulties. You have to deal with serious problems at a personal level as well as a professional level . . . that can be hard, especially if you are asking people to do things that are uncomfortable. On the other hand, people trust you already, even little children who know you because they go to school with your kids, and that makes it easier. (Cited in Bowles, 2010: 16–17)

THEORY AND POLICY CONTEXT OF THE DISABILITY FIELD

Since the United Nations International Year of Disabled People (1981), people with disabilities, their families and supporters have struggled to transform the disability field. Initially a policy backwater dominated by the medical model in which people with disabilities were treated at best as victims of individual tragedy, the disability field is now recognised as an international human rights priority, and disability itself is regarded as a matter of social inclusion. Today official definitions of disability emphasise the role of environmental barriers, including attitudes, so that disability is understood as a multi-dimensional social construct—as much an issue of social justice and human rights as of physical or mental impairment (AIHW, 2009a: 139). Coming from a shared ethical base prioritising human rights and social justice (AASW, 2010), the disability field should be a natural place for social work.

By signing the UN Convention on the Rights of Persons with Disabilities (United Nations, 2008), Australia has committed to principles of equality of citizenship for people with disabilities, and 'mainstreaming' their access to all levels of services such as transport, health care, education and employment opportunities. The eight principles laid down by the Convention resonate strongly with social work principles, and revolve around respect, diversity, participation, inclusion and equality (see United Nations, 2008, 2010). Australia's Draft National Disability Strategy, aimed at implementing the principles of the UN Convention in Australia, is the result of national consultations during 2008–09, summarised in the *Shut Out* report cited above (National People with Disabilities and Carers Council, 2009). Based on a whole-of-life and whole-of-government approach, it recommends policy developments in six areas:

1 inclusive and accessible communities
2 rights protection, justice and legislation
3 economic security
4 personal and community support
5 learning and skills, and
6 health and well-being (see Council of Australian Governments, 2010).

The third plank of recent disability policy in Australia is the National Disability Agreement, which came into effect on 1 January 2009 (see COAG, 2009). A summary of the key features of this agreement, with its focus on specialist services for people with disability, ten priority areas for reform and 'person-centred' services, is found in the chapter 'Disability Services' in *Australia's Welfare* (AIHW, 2009a). This policy framework is underpinned by rights-based federal and state legislation, including the various Disability Services Acts and the *Disability Discrimination Act* 1992.

Despite all these policy advances, disability remains a site of struggle for social inclusion. Research shows that efforts to include people with disabilities as citizens in mainstream society are plagued with difficulties (e.g. see Bigby, 2008; Clement & Bigby, 2009).

SERVICE-DELIVERY MODELS AND METHODS OF PRACTICE IN THE DISABILITY FIELD IN RURAL AND REGIONAL AREAS

Whether rural or urban based, during the twentieth century many parents of people with disabilities worked to set up their own services for family members with disabilities, often with the support of service groups. For example, Rotary instigated Northcott Disability Services (Northcott Disability Services, 2011), which began in 1929 in Sydney, and Wagga Apex Club and Wagga Jaycees supported

Kurrajong Waratah (Kurrajong Waratah, 2011), which began in 1957 in Wagga Wagga, New South Wales. From small beginnings, these groups grew to become non-government services, often with a management structure that included parents of people with disabilities. With the rise of the disability rights movement and the various Acts discussed above, having people with disabilities contribute to and participate in the management of their own services as part of their citizenship rights and responsibilities became a funding requirement for most services during the late 1980s and 1990s.

Prior to the 1990s, many people with disabilities living in small towns, and their families, had to move to larger centres to access services. Those who stayed did so with very little support. However, in small towns during the late 1980s and early 1990s, in response to policy moves based in notions of rights and citizenship such as 'ageing in place', and despite the documented lack of resources in comparison to the larger regional and urban areas, a surprising array of small services emerged for people with disabilities. In West Wyalong, a group home for supported accommodation, a coffee shop, and gardening and recycling businesses employing people with disabilities were established. The local management committees running these services struggled to find members with the expertise needed to deal with ever-changing urban-based bureaucratic and legislative requirements to maintain funding. They were also acutely aware of the changing needs of the ageing group of carers and people with disabilities, who increasingly did not fit with the existing service models.

Other aspects of the disability field in West Wyalong include an Access Sub-committee, chaired by a social worker, formed in 1999 to advise council on how to improve access throughout the Bland Shire. This group developed an access policy and plan for the shire, as well as community access awards and an access incentive scheme, offering funding to improve access to premises for local businesses and community services. Another model of disability service delivery to small towns such as West Wyalong involves having visiting professionals from the New South Wales Health Department and other state departments, who are based in larger centres, visit small towns on a regular or sometimes ad hoc basis to provide much-needed therapy and early intervention services. Known as the 'hub and spoke' model, this is a common way of providing services across a large region, particularly in rural areas.

In 2002, the employment services in West Wyalong merged with a much larger provider of disability services, Kurrajong Waratah, based

150 kilometres away in Wagga Wagga. Reflecting the shift from the medical/charity model to the rights model, Kurrajong Waratah's cafe changed its name from SPINS (Special People in Need of Support) to Cafe Peckish. In response to discussions with local people, Kurrajong Waratah also undertook to establish a day service for older people with disabilities who could not meet the requirements for the employment services, but wanted some way to participate in the community. Skills Options West Wyalong opened its doors in 2006.

In 2004, West Wyalong's group home, Marashel, also moved under the umbrella of Kurrajong Waratah Disability Services. Partly, the increasingly complex and detailed accountability requirements of the various funding bodies, together with insurance, staffing needs and other considerations, were becoming too onerous for small voluntary management committees. In addition, it was recognised that Kurrajong Waratah, with its larger resources, could provide a stronger and more sustainable professional base for services for people with disabilities and the staff who worked with them in the West Wyalong community. A parent representative from West Wyalong was appointed to the Kurrajong Waratah Board. Disability services in other small towns in the region have made similar decisions, with disability services from the towns of Leeton and Narrandera also merging with Kurrajong Waratah in recent years.

Kurrajong Waratah itself was initially established in 1957 to provide services for children with developmental disabilities in Wagga Wagga. Since those early days, this organisation has expanded to become an auspice for a wide range of services offering disability services across the Riverina Murray region of New South Wales. These include early childhood intervention, employment, accommodation, day activity services, leisure, respite and support for people with disabilities and their families. The Riverina Murray region covers an area encompassing 26 local government areas and 19.2 per cent of New South Wales—similar to the size of Tasmania.

From this brief overview of some of the service models for people with disabilities and their families in rural areas, it is obvious that all the methods of practice used by social workers would be valuable in this field, particularly in small towns, and rural and regional areas. However, given the comparative scarcity of resources in small towns, it is most likely that social workers will be involved in various forms of community assessment, development and management in addition to clinical roles, as they strive to enable access to services for as many people as possible.

One of the features of the social model is the principle that professional relationships must be partnerships, based on mutual respect and shared goals. Social workers and other professionals are expected to be colleagues and allies with people with disabilities as they confront the barriers (both attitudinal and environmental) that make their lives so much more difficult than those of people without disabilities. The traditional 'one-up' relationship of the professional knowing what is best for the client is not accepted in this field. Instead, clients, their families/advocates and professionals alike must be active participants in planning, implementing and evaluating the interventions they devise.

CASE STUDY: INTERLINK

InterLink is a division of Kurrajong Waratah which provides short-term case management to older parent carers with the care responsibility of a family member with disability living at home with them. To be eligible for service, carers of people with disabilities must live in the Riverina Murray Region, and be 60 years of age or older for non-Indigenous carers or 45 years of age or older for Indigenous carers (in recognition of the shorter life span and greater level of disadvantage experienced by Indigenous people).

Initially established as a two-year pilot program in 2007, InterLink aims to provide short-term support and assistance to ageing carers across the region, including linking people with mainstream and specialist services such as home modifications, home care, respite care (or a planned break for the carer) and planning for emergency care and long-term future care for the person with a disability. The ten Key Result Areas specified in the InterLink funding contract from ADHC (NSW Department of Human Services, 2008) include that the service should locate and provide support to hidden carers, focus on including Indigenous carers, and respectfully involve all older parent carers (clients) in decision-making for their future.

In practice, InterLink staff connect families with existing resources within their area, and develop individualised emergency care and future care plans. Emergency care plans are usually kept on the refrigerator or in an obvious place in the home for times of emergency such as when carers need to be hospitalised. Emergency care plans detail care arrangements, as well as daily requirements and routines for the person with a disability who will need to be cared for by someone else during the emergency. The InterLink service also includes developing longer-term future care plans with carers for the time when the ageing carers can no longer continue in their role. In addition, InterLink offers a needs-based 'carers assistance package', which is a one-off payment for goods and services to improve or sustain the current care arrangements, as well as access to a free-call emergency number for all older parent carers. Thus social workers working as coordinators require good assessment skills. They need to assess not only the carers' needs, but also the environmental resources and barriers that will help or hinder carers in their role and thus enable the person with a disability to remain in their family and community. Skills of advocacy, brokerage and sometimes community and service development are also required. In 2010, InterLink had 250 clients on its books. Not all are active clients, as the service is short term (Steve Jaques, pers. comm., 8 February 2011), but they are followed up every six months to see whether anything in the care arrangements has changed or needs changing.

During 2010, two social work students evaluated older parent carers' satisfaction with InterLink (Finlay & Dwyer, 2010). A notable finding was that 44 per cent of respondents had been found by InterLink staff rather than being referred or seeking service, thus demonstrating InterLink's success in locating hidden carers. Further, whereas only 30 per cent of respondents reported having enough help before their contact with InterLink, over 70 per cent reported that they now had enough help. Overwhelmingly, these ageing carers were satisfied with InterLink's services (96 per cent), commenting on the practical support for wheelchairs, ramps and hot water systems, as well as information and support; one respondent said that 'They have given me the help that no other service has provided. I know that I can call anytime if I need assistance' (respondent number 72, quoted in Finlay & Dwyer, 2010: 33). These kinds of results echo the positive experiences people with disabilities and their carers can have in small towns and rural areas, also reported by Jessica Smith at the beginning of this chapter. However, respondents also consistently requested longer-term contact with InterLink, including more respite, support and linkages to other services. Clearly the short-term case management model mandated by the funding body is not the right model for ageing carers living with ageing sons and daughters with disabilities in small towns and rural and remote areas.

Reflective questions

- How would you approach and engage with ageing older parent carers who have never before received any support for their adult son or daughter with a disability, to offer the kinds of support discussed in the case study above?
- Considering the results of the evaluation study of InterLink, make a list of possible key contacts (organisations and key contact roles) in small towns that would help you to work effectively with people with disabilities and their supporters.
- How would you go about advocating for ageing people with disabilities in small towns and their carers within the social model?
- How could you work with the high levels of social capital implied by the quote that began this chapter, in order to assist people with disabilities to overcome the barriers they face? List some strategies to engage the strengths of small towns.

SUMMARY

The disability field in small towns is a challenging and rewarding area for social workers. Notwithstanding the documented barriers, people with disabilities in small towns can experience high levels of support and encouragement, as illustrated in Jessica Smith's quote. The story of InterLink demonstrates that social and welfare workers in small towns really do make a positive difference in people's lives.

RECOMMENDED READING

Policy context of the disability field in Australia

Australian Institute of Health and Welfare (AIHW) (2009) Disability and disability services. In AIHW, *Australia's Welfare 2009*. AIHW, Canberra.

Bullock, S. (2010) Whose health? How population groups vary. In AIHW, *Australia's Health 2010*, AIHW, Canberra.

Social work in the disability field

Bigby, C. & Frawley, P. (2010) *Social Work Practice and Intellectual Disability*. Palgrave Macmillan, Basingstoke.

Bowles, W. (2005) Social work and people with disabilities. In M. Alston & J. McKinnon (eds), *Social Work Fields of Practice*, 2nd edn. Oxford University Press, Melbourne.

ACKNOWLEDGEMENT

The author is most grateful to Steve Jaques, Chief Executive Officer of Kurrajong Waratah, for reading drafts of this chapter, providing information, comments and insights, and for permission to quote from unpublished research evaluating the InterLink Service.

8

DEALING WITH VIOLENCE: FAMILIES LIVING IN RURAL SETTLEMENTS

Robyn Mason

CHAPTER OBJECTIVES

- To describe aspects of social work practice in the field of violence against women, informed by research, policy and knowledge about service delivery.
- To focus on potential issues facing social work, including immigration experiences and drug and alcohol use.
- To identify the impact of specific location and employment factors on family and community life in mining communities.
- To identify relevant anti-oppressive social work practice approaches in this setting.

INTRODUCTION

This chapter has a focus on a particular field of practice, violence against women, and a particular location, remote mining communities. In these places, residents confront challenges due to location, employment arrangements, gender roles, cultural difference and use of leisure. In Australia, since white settlement, mining has been a major economic activity. There is a history of ebb and flow in the industry: new mines and new surrounding communities are opened up, thrive for a short period and then close when the ore is depleted or when it is no longer profitable to continue mining. The uncertainty and impermanent nature of the industry have an impact on the livelihood experiences of residents, whether they are directly or indirectly involved in mining. Mining is also firmly entrenched in the stereotypical view of outback Australia as a tough, masculine environment where mateship is paramount and where women, if present at all, have clearly defined minor roles.

Mining communities feature leisure activities that encourage men to spend time together outside working hours (Collis, 1999; Gibson, 1994). Rosters conducive to streamlining production, utilising long-distance commuting and shiftwork, mean that women often experience isolation (Iverson & Maguire, 2000), solely caring for children and managing households for long periods. These working arrangements have been dubbed 'divorce rosters' by women who experience conflict when men's loyalties seem to be torn between the family at home and the 'family' of workmates (Gibson, 1994). Managing the consequent impact on relationships, family life and community engagement is a serious social challenge, worthy of social work attention.

VIOLENCE AGAINST WOMEN

Violence against women is now high on the public policy agenda in Australia, but this was not always the case. The women's movement of the late twentieth century succeeded in exposing crimes of physical, sexual and emotional violence perpetrated against women and children, in the home by intimate partners, and in institutions and the community by men outside the family, including clergy and men in other trusted positions. The formal, funded service sector responding to these crimes, run mainly by women volunteers in the 1970s, evolved in the 1980s. These services, supporting women escaping violence and women who have survived sexual assault, are small and under-resourced, and coverage in rural and remote Australia is inadequate.

In this chapter I use the term 'violence against women' to mean all those categories of interpersonal violence experienced by women and perpetrated by men, including physical, emotional and psychological abuse, as well as all the forms of sexual violence experienced by women and perpetrated by men, including sexual assault, rape and harassment. In the field, terms may be used deliberately to denote a particular ideology, such as 'family violence', preferred by some Aboriginal community members, or 'domestic violence', preferred by some funding bodies. Sometimes these terms are used interchangeably. 'Intimate partner violence' is another term to further clarify the nature of the abuse. In the sector, services may be known as domestic violence support services, women's support services, women's refuges, domestic violence outreach services, rape crisis centres or sexual assault support services. In discussing violence against women, workers in the sexual assault field have been at pains to point out that most women reporting domestic violence have also been victims of sexual violence. The service sector, historically divided into specialist domestic violence agencies and sexual assault support agencies, has tended to classify women's experience in unhelpful ways, perpetuating the artificial dividing up of women's lives and thereby not always offering the most appropriate service response.

Violence against women in rural Australia is not well understood. The Women's Services Network (WESNET) (2000) reviewed the available research and identified a number of gaps, including the need for more information about service models in rural areas, and about the extent and nature of violence experienced by groups of women in rural and remote areas. There is a view that there are particular features of the rural culture that increase women's vulnerability to violence and discourage help-seeking (Wendt, 2009), or that the multiple connections among rural residents make it difficult for women to report or escape from violence (Rawsthorne, 2008). Research has also documented specific factors in rural and remote environments that hinder women's right to live free from violence. These have been summarised as: isolation, both geographic and economic; the presence of firearms; a lack of access to legal protections, including confidentiality and privacy; inconsistent police responses and reluctance to report to police; fear of more violence or death for themselves and their children if they seek help; poor access to services, lack of services or inappropriate urban service models; and financial insecurity, exacerbated by complex financial arrangements regarding family farm ownership (WESNET, 2000). All of these factors, as well as the stigma and shame attached to formal help-seeking in a small community, a lack of resources, poverty and distance, have also been noted by women's service providers in rural Australia as specific to rural areas (Mason, 2007).

Turning to the issue of violence against women in mining communities, there is a similar gap in the available research. The WESNET (2000) review mentions women in mining communities as a specific group but lists only one reference to research. Characteristics of mining communities are listed as barriers for women experiencing violence to seek help or to end a violent relationship, including a lack of community cohesion because of fly-in/fly-out arrangements and transience; isolation from family and supports; limited employment opportunities for women; little choice about housing; and an inadequate service sector (WESNET, 2000).

A recent contribution from Queensland (Nancarrow et al., 2009) sheds more light on what is actually occurring for women in mining cultures. Researchers surveyed 532 women in a mining area in Central Queensland, to examine the nature and prevalence of intimate partner abuse. They found that these women did not experience more intimate partner abuse than women across Australia generally, despite the view expressed by some human service workers that rates were higher in that region. They concluded that 'mining cultures had no demonstrable association with women's experience of most forms of abuse' (Nancarrow et al., 2009: 5). However, it is worth reiterating the key findings of the study, in order to provide a context for the discussion to follow. The study found that abuse of women was more prevalent in de facto relationships rather than marital relationships, and where partners had been together for less than five years rather than fifteen years or more. The women more likely to experience socio-psychological abuse were those in relationships less than five years old; those who were mostly responsible for children; those in de facto rather than marital partnerships; those under 30 years of age; and those with no access to a joint bank account. Women were at increased risk of socio-psychological abuse if their partners had grown up in a mining area or had limited education. Women with children living at home were at greater risk than women without children living at home. For physical and other non-physical abuse,

> women in de facto relationships, women aged less than 30 years, women solely or mostly responsible for children, women with joint debt up to $100,000 and women with no access to a joint bank account had increased risk of physical and non-physical forms of abuse. (Nancarrow et al., 2009: 4)

The study found that consumption of alcohol ('risky drinking'), smoking and the use of other drugs were factors for men and women affected by violence, with men's use of cannabis the greatest risk for intimate partner abuse.

Some research suggests that the violence and cruelty associated with the workplace culture of mining towns spills over into the leisure and domestic spheres (Hogg & Carrington, 2006). Service providers in one town reported 'cruel initiation rituals and deplorable work conditions' that had an impact on how men related to others outside work, and especially on their control of wives and children (Hogg & Carrington, 2006: 178). The town under study experienced high rates of violence between men as well as violence against women, and high rates of alcohol consumption. A further important factor to consider is the significant impact of violence on women's mental health, demonstrated in increased evidence of severe psychological symptoms and depression for women exposed to intimate partner abuse (Nancarrow et al., 2009). Even more concerning, however, is the finding that the unique nature of mining communities and the work arrangements experienced in the mining industry contribute to psychiatric illness in women whose partners work in the mines, because of the strain placed on relationships (Sharma & Rees, 2007).

REMOTE MINING COMMUNITIES: THE CONTEXT

In a broad, structural sense, the stressors outlined above are linked with the consequences of globalisation and rural restructuring, where some places grow while others decline in response to the vagaries of international markets. One consequence of these global changes has been the growth of single-industry towns such as mining towns in remote places. These settlements are often constructed or created because of the mining resource, and have an air of artificiality or transience, without the strong connections among people that we might expect to see in other non-metropolitan settings. It is worth identifying the features of remote communities and what makes them different from urban communities. Roderick D. Iverson and Catherine Maguire (2000: 808) list six features of remote communities:

1 difficult physical environment
2 high economic and social cost involved in the exploitation of natural resources
3 unattractive places in which to live
4 expensive basic services
5 total population is restricted to a level required for the operation of the resource activity and is typically unbalanced and highly mobile, and

6 population is often considered to be deprived because of its isolation.

Working in the mining industry is said to be an attractive option because of money and employment opportunities, the chance to increase one's standard of living, a better climate and an opportunity to join friends or family in the mining community (Iverson & Maguire, 2000). In Australia, tales from the resource-rich states suggest that working in mining means hard manual work in high-paying jobs, located in frontier towns where there are few amenities and where a hard-drinking culture prevails. For some Aboriginal communities, agreements with mining ventures may result in royalty payments as compensation for loss of land. Most Aboriginal people located in or near mining communities, however, experience displacement from country and exclusion from the livelihood opportunities offered to non-Aboriginal people. In this sense, the mining boom represents a further lost opportunity for the First Australians to share in the nation's prosperity.[1] Indeed, Aboriginal people are noticeably 'marginal or absent' (Hogg & Carrington, 2006: 200) from discourses about rural cultures in Australia, as if they occupy a parallel universe. Similarly, partly as a response to global economic restructuring, women from Asia began to arrive in the Pilbara region of Western Australia more than two decades ago, with many experiencing isolation and economic marginalisation (Reeve, 1994). Again, we hear little about their experience. There is anecdotal evidence from remote human service workers that women—especially women from Asia—are at risk of sexual violence and sex slavery. There has been one such case detected in a mining town in Far North Queensland, where a couple has been convicted of slavery of a Filipino woman lured to Australia for a sham marriage (Schwarten, 2010).

The perception of mining towns as tough, all-male enclaves is one that some mining companies and health and human service workers are attempting to change, opting instead to promote the view of a mining town as family-friendly (Culf, 2009). A welcome program for new residents in Roxby Downs, South Australia, is an attempt to respond to the growth in population, especially the influx of

---

[1] A partnership between Fortescue Metals and the Commonwealth Government (Fortescue Metals Group, 2010) aims to increase employment opportunities for Aboriginal people in the mining industry. For more information, go to <www.fmgl.com.au/irm/Community/index.html>.

families with young children. Features of the Roxby Downs community include the temporary status of most people, with 75 per cent of the population staying for five years, and a monocultural profile, where most residents are Australian-born and English-speaking, although new residents from other cultural backgrounds are beginning to arrive. Their needs are for specialist support to address isolation and the risk of depression. The welcome program was one outcome of a community consultation that developed a community plan to address identified needs such as loneliness and depression, poor access to health services and a lack of connectedness. The program is a partnership between the mining company and the health service. Reading between the lines, the program attempts to address the characteristics of mining communities outlined above, which facilitate a culture that promotes violence—although the issue of violence is not mentioned in information promoting the program. Joanne Culf (2009) concludes that:

> Building social capital is a key characteristic of the Big Warm Welcome in our communities; it is about being more than a resource. It is about enhancing people's sense of belonging, community cooperation, trust and positive participation in community activities. (2009: 46)

SERVICE DELIVERY

Research informs us that the provision of support services in rural and remote communities is constrained by factors such as distance, visibility, a lack of referral options for workers, poor access to specialist workers, inadequate professional development opportunities for workers, concerns about privacy and confidentiality, and the blurring of personal and professional boundaries (Green, 2003). Services are often generic, addressing broad health and family support needs, rather than specialist agencies. A services directory from the Pilbara in Western Australia, for example, includes a small number of services for women escaping violence under the broad heading of child and family services (West Pilbara Communities for Children, 2010). Locating women's support services under generic categories in this way serves to hide the gendered nature of violence; as reported earlier, maintaining silence about violence is a feature of some rural communities (Rawsthorne, 2008; Wendt, 2009).

Addressing violence against women, service models across Australia include early intervention programs targeting workers in generalist services such as police, hospitals and schools; prevention programs operating in schools and sporting clubs, with a focus on building healthy and respectful relationships; public advocacy and community education campaigns about violence and its impact; crisis response services providing immediate medical support, safe accommodation and crisis counselling; and medium and longer-term service provision, including counselling, groupwork and opportunities for social action. One would expect all of these problems to be magnified in a mining community, where the population is thrown together to meet employment needs, services are few or non-existent and there is little formal or informal support for women seeking assistance.

POLICY CONTEXT

As social workers, we are informed, and sometimes constrained, by the policy context in the particular fields in which we operate. The policies driving programs and services in the violence-against-women field are making a shift away from crisis and direct practice approaches (although there is a recognition that women will always require crisis and therapeutic support), to the development of programs aimed at preventing or reducing violence. The Commonwealth and several states have begun to articulate and resource prevention strategies, including media campaigns and school programs. Similarly, social work practice in mining communities cannot ignore the abuse of alcohol and other drugs, so social workers need to increase their knowledge about current trends in that field. Harm minimisation has become a common approach in the drug treatment field, while the Commonwealth government has put resources into a national alcohol strategy, mainly targeting young people's binge drinking (Department of Health and Ageing, 2010). Understanding and responding to the policy context, and positioning ourselves to influence policy, means that we can access resources for our service users, as well as ensure that policy-makers are informed about the lived experience of the people we serve.

AN ANTI-OPPRESSIVE APPROACH

How best can we underpin our practice in an environment such as the one I have described? An anti-oppressive approach is one that acknowledges important and fundamental principles of social work, such as respect for persons, social justice and a non-judgemental stance. It is therefore useful in a situation where people face barriers because they may not be seen to be part of the mainstream or dominant group. In recent times we have come to a clearer understanding of how these barriers operate and their impact on people. Those most likely to experience forms of discrimination present differently from the dominant culture in terms of race, gender, ethnicity, ability, age, class and, I would argue, location. What these groups experience is a form of oppression, one that is not always easily identified or visible. In Australia, for example, we have established institutions and processes that operationalise our stated commitment to a free and fair society; a rule of law that protects and upholds our right to live safely and to seek redress when wronged; political and social citizenship rights; a stable democratic system of government; and protections for workers fought for and defended over many decades by working people and trade unions. Nonetheless, there is no doubt that not everyone in Australia benefits equally from these arrangements. Aboriginal people, for example, experience unacceptably high levels of unemployment and incarceration in our prisons; one in three women is a victim of men's violence; asylum seekers are demonised and held in desert detention camps; reports of child abuse are rising exponentially; the number of homeless people is on the increase. Oppression is also present, if not so visible, in the way access to education is restricted, in how health services are distributed, in where the best jobs are available.

Oppression, then, may be 'structurally systemic, covert or hidden, and unintentional' (Mullaly, 2002: 40). Mullaly argues that oppression is most effective if oppressors and the oppressed are unaware of how oppression operates:

> When people perceive their situation as natural and inevitable, and there is an illusion of freedom and opportunity, no other weapons are necessary to defend and legitimate unjust ways of life that benefit the privileged groups at the expense of the oppressed groups. (Mullaly, 2002: 40)

Oppression is built into our institutions and our social relations: we contribute to it and are victims of it as we go about our lives. As social workers, we are obliged to analyse these processes so that we are aware of our own contribution to oppression and begin to understand how our service users may be experiencing this phenomenon.

A useful way to think about anti-oppressive practice is to see intervention operating on three levels: the personal, the cultural and the structural (Thompson, 2006). At the personal level, we will be concerned with how service users see themselves and the psychological impact of violence, such as self-blame, guilt, a lack of confidence, or depression. At this level, the personal experience of women experiencing violence is linked with the political, so that invisible pillars of oppression are exposed. In practice terms, this may mean empowering women so that they can name their experience as violence, making available to them the language they need to do so and affirming with them that their experience is shared in common with other women in similar situations. As Mullaly states, the emphasis is on 'the sameness and common ground of the oppressed persons' (Mullaly, 2002: 181).

The cultural level, according to Neil Thompson (2006), is where we see the influence of society in the beliefs we hold about social arrangements. In terms of violence against women, there are powerful influences operating to perpetuate cultural myths about women and men, advanced through the media, education and the persistence of gender stereotypes. To counteract these influences, Mullaly (2002) encourages the celebration of alternative cultures as a way of challenging and resisting the dominant culture. Good examples of action at the cultural level to challenge the dominant culture about violence against women include media campaigns that promote alternative views of masculinity (such as the 'Real men don't hit women' campaign), and the annual recognition of violence against women on 25 November, now known as White Ribbon Day. Programs and events like these are examples of resistance to the dominant culture. They represent an alternative way of seeing and interpreting the world, and they confront stereotypes. Social workers can address oppression at the cultural level by celebrating alternative cultures, challenging dominant discourses and confronting stereotypes (for example, about Filipino 'mail-order brides' or what constitutes real masculinity).

The cultural dimensions of oppression, Thompson (2006: 23) reminds us, are embedded in the structural level, defined as the web of 'social divisions and the power relations which maintain them'. At this level, the social worker addresses change in institutions, policies, laws and systems that serve to perpetuate oppression. Working in the anti-violence field, examples of action at the structural level include advocacy for family violence law reform undertaken by women working collectively across services, government and the justice system, or work by women to address violence in a comprehensive or whole-of-government approach. Another example of a structural challenge to oppression that also confronts cultural beliefs is the violence-prevention program in schools that operates in some Australian states. These approaches have Commonwealth government support, and are seen to be a way of changing behaviour over the long term (National Council to Reduce Violence Against Women and their Children, 2009).

Social workers can also address oppression at the structural level by supporting the formation of new social movements and building coalitions of workers, organisations and service users to effect change. Social workers need to get political: whether we are members of political parties or politically active in local communities, standing for political office, joining regional bodies or professional associations, our voices need to be heard.

CASE STUDY

Virginia, aged 30, is married to Brad, aged 48, a mine worker. They live in Minetown, a coal-mining community with a population of about 4000, situated 300 kilometres inland from the city of Mackay in Queensland. Brad works four twelve-hour shifts over four days, then has four days off. Shift rosters vary from day, afternoon and night shifts and workers have one weekend off each month. Brad, who left school after Year 10, grew up and worked in a coal-mining area in another state, but when that mine closed down he moved to Queensland in search of employment. Approaching 40 years of age and with little time for socialising, Brad had limited success in connecting with local women so, on the advice of a married friend, joined an internet club specialising in finding Asian women interested in marrying Australian men. There he made contact with Virginia, then in her early twenties, a new graduate with a marketing degree who was living in Manila and working in a casual job at an advertising agency to support her parents and younger siblings. Virginia sought the legitimacy and opportunities that marriage to an Australian man would bring, and after two enjoyable face-to-face meetings, in Manila and in Brisbane, they were married eight years ago. They now have two children—Mark, aged six and Bella, aged three. Although Virginia has made some friendships in Minetown, especially with other Filipina women through attendance at church, she often feels isolated and lonely, spending a lot of time as the 'sole parent' because of Brad's work demands. She is very keen to return to her career, but Brad does not believe that married women should work while their children are young. She is also concerned that Brad does not give her sufficient funds to run the household: he controls the finances, pays the accounts and makes the decisions about purchasing expensive items such as whitegoods and furnishings. She has asked him several times for more money for groceries and clothes for the children, but he has become very angry each time, shouting abuse at her in front of the children, accusing her of sending all the money to her family in the Philippines, and storming out of the house. More recently, he has been spending more of his leisure time with workmates at the pub or at the golf course. Other women say the same is happening for them, so Virginia accepts that this is the way things are in the town and that there is little she can do about it. She tries now to have the house quiet and the children asleep or playing outside when he is at home, where he spends most of his time drinking and playing computer games in the living room.

Mark has just started school and is displaying some behaviours that appear to be limiting his learning. The class teacher has asked to see Virginia and Brad to discuss referring Mark to the visiting school psychologist, who comes to Minetown once a month. When Virginia sought Brad's support to attend the school meeting with her, Brad lashed out verbally, blaming her for Mark's 'so-called learning problems', and threatening to find someone else to raise his children. Virginia mentioned this incident to Gloria, a Filipina friend who works in the supermarket. Gloria has offered to accompany Virginia to the community health centre for a duty appointment with the part-time social worker.

Reflective questions

Exercise 1
Discuss in class or note down your responses to the following.
- Critically reflect on your reactions to the Virginia and Brad story. Are there features of the story that make you feel

uncomfortable? Are there some issues you would prefer not to address? What might be the reasons for your reluctance?

- Working with Virginia and Brad, how would you address the oppression experienced by each of them at the personal level, the cultural level and the structural level? Try to suggest practical strategies that you might apply at each level.
- What would be your plan for future work with Virginia, Brad and the children?

Exercise 2
- Imagine you are the social planner at the shire of Minetown, and that the council has asked you to address the perceived lack of social connectedness in the town. Draw up two columns, one headed 'Community Well-being Strategy' and the other headed 'Supporting Evidence'.
- Use the first column to outline the features of and processes for your proposed Community Well-being Strategy—for example, run a community consultation about violence; complete an audit of available services; address excess alcohol consumption, and so on.
- Use the second column to list the evidence that supports each step, such as the research about violence against women in mining towns, current policy about alcohol use, the application of anti-oppressive social work practice principles, and so on.
- You may need to do some further research about some of these issues in order to complete the 'evidence' column.

SUMMARY

This chapter has described aspects of practice relevant to the field of violence against women, informed by research findings, current policy and knowledge about service delivery models, especially in rural Australia. The context was a specific location—remote mining communities—where there were unique impacts of location, employment conditions, livelihood constraints and community cohesion. The chapter identified some potential impacts of these specific location and employment factors on family and community life. The case study focused on how the issue of violence against women might be played out in a mining community, highlighting the migrant experience and excessive alcohol use. An anti-oppressive social work practice approach was presented as a relevant response to the issues arising in the case study.

RECOMMENDED READING

Cunneen, C. & Stubbs, J. (2007) *Migration, Political Economy and Violence Against Women: The post-immigration experiences of Filipino women in Australia.* Legal Studies Research Paper 07/25, University of Sydney Law School, Sydney.

National Council to Reduce Violence Against Women and Their Children (2009) *Time for Action: The National Council's plan for Australia to reduce violence against women and their children, 2009–2021.* National Council to Reduce Violence Against Women and Their Children, Canberra.

Roces, N. (2003) Sisterhood is local: Filipino women in Mount Isa. In N. Piper & N. Roces (eds), *Wife or Worker? Asian women and migration.* Rowman and Littlefield, Lanham, MD, pp. 73–100.

Rose, D. & Farrow, J. (2009) Perspectives on drug use. In M. Connolly & L. Harms (eds), *Social Work Contexts and Practice*, 2nd edn. Oxford University Press, Melbourne, pp. 248–61.

9

ANALYSING CRIMINALISATION IN RURAL COMMUNITY CONTEXTS

David McCallum

CHAPTER OBJECTIVES

- To identify stresses of rural family life that underpin violence.
- To describe the processes that lead to the criminalising of families.
- To examine positive service delivery responses and opportunities to reduce violence.
- To identify specific cultural factors in rural settings that support non-violence.

INTRODUCTION

Most of Australia's prisons and detention centres are located in rural areas, and rates of incarceration have increased significantly in recent times. The 'prisonisation' of Australia, although not as visible as in the United States, has continued unabated for the past two decades. Since the mid-1980s, the rate of male imprisonment has doubled and the rate of female imprisonment has trebled. Rates of recidivism are also high, particularly for Indigenous women, of whom 63 per cent return to prison compared with 38 per cent for non-Indigenous women. In addition, the majority (two-thirds) of offenders managed by correctional services in Australia are serving community-based orders, which often involves strong family and community engagement with the offender. The vast majority of prisoners come from disadvantaged families, and the most disadvantaged group—Indigenous Australians—has a rate of imprisonment seventeen times higher than the non-Indigenous population. Indigenous young people in Victoria are imprisoned at 22 times the rate of non-Indigenous youth (Australian Institute of Criminology, 2010). These events are significant because welfare policies and practices have a major bearing on the resilience of families under social and economic pressures. Prison stands at one end of the spectrum of endpoints, stronger inclusive communities at the other. Personal and institutional violence are often at the core of imprisonment rates, and rural communities in Australia are experiencing some of the highest rates of violence in the country.

This chapter focuses on family violence, and discusses the ways in which welfare interventions are critical to reducing criminalisation and the pathways leading to prisons. This is especially important for the life trajectories of rural individuals and families under stress. There is abundant evidence that levels of interpersonal violence are higher in rural than non-rural areas, and that much of this violence is perpetrated by men against women and children. People experiencing stress often find a light at the end of the tunnel through community strengthening and engagement. Participatory approaches are especially important in building ordinary people's capacity to analyse and transform their lives, and provide a practical means to facilitate empowerment and build community resilience. This chapter reports on research that tends to confirm a sociological truism: that it is social processes rather than individual choices which most often determine the life chances open to people. Here we look at some of the research on interventions in families that can increase people's options and explore how rural life can help or hinder empowerment, or alternatively can lead to criminalising family members, particularly women and young people.

It should be noted that social and economic circumstances explain people's resort to violent acts, rather than explanations like human nature or genetics, and that underlying stresses lead to interpersonal tensions, not the reverse. Before sifting out some of the elements in the rural environment that underpin family violence in particular, it is necessary to explain briefly the theoretical orientation of the research approaches reviewed in the chapter.

In the last decade, much of rural and regional Australia has endured the crippling effects of a global economic downturn along with drought or massive floods (and sometimes both). Social supports for the people affected by these events have been placed under severe strain. Some traditional rural industries have fared badly during this period, although one exception is prisons and detention centres often located in or near rural centres that provide livelihoods in a range of employment and services. Unlike some rural industries, prisons are booming.

GOVERNING FAMILIES

Some recent research on prisons, the welfare system, and families and children under stress has approached the interrelations between these social problems through a study of 'mentalities of governing', or 'governmentality'—how ways of thinking and acting on problems come into being over time, taking on a particular shape and in turn informing the way we manage these problems (Foucault, 1991). Here we want to look at examples of research that focus on mentalities of governing the interrelations around families. Mentalities of governing also assume that our present social relations are always mediated by contexts arising from social relations in the past. I draw on this approach to examine some key issues in criminalisation that have led to the large increases in prison populations throughout Australia, and have also brought rural families and communities into sharp focus as a site of governing.

Social work forms part of the social expertise deployed since the early part of the twentieth century to promote family well-being. Although not directly coterminous with the development of the welfare state, the emerging apparatus for intervening in families accompanied the strengthening of institutions like hospitals, philanthropy and policing—primarily to support families to govern themselves (McCallum, 2009). This view can be contrasted with the social control aspects of the profession, which highlight the policing role of social work in its management of parental behaviours in the context of its statutory powers to recommend the removal of children through the courts. The main problem with social control theory is that it assumes individuals are passive victims of interventions, and that power relations involve top-down actions by those who possess power on to those who do not. Modern forms of power, by contrast, tend to be productive rather than repressive, and engage with individuals and groups in ways that incite them to adopt social norms. The approach taken here is to view social work's relationships to families in terms of resilience-building through primary prevention programs, along with a focus on forms of governing that emphasise self-regulation and 'care of the self' (Foucault, 2008).

Jacques Donzelot's (1979) concept of 'psy-techniques' is an important one—a non-coercive correction in the family where power takes the form of encouraging families to seek to align their conduct to social norms. In the case of threats to liberal society, the state may intervene to 'apply the norm'. Law and legal process is also present insofar as intervention in the so-called private sphere of the family is a site of tension within liberal forms of government. Donzelot in fact points to the paradox of a liberalised and more autonomous family, while at the same time 'the strangle hold of a tutelary authority tightens around the poor family' (1979: 108). Here, Donzelot points to social norms often identified with dominant social groups that come to be imposed upon subordinate groups. In turn, the health and well-being of an entire population come to be linked to the development of modern family forms. Theories of governing along these lines assume that historically reinforced distinctions between public and private allow central forms of governing to step back from interfering and permit families to be sites of governing in themselves. Liberalism is, after all, concerned with the uneconomic aspects of 'too much governing', and that includes too much 'public' interference in the 'private' sphere of the family. The term 'governing through the family' refers to a withdrawal of central governing involvement with the minutiae of everyday life, while at the same time 'governing at a distance' to ensure it can intervene in the family if necessary.

We can observe immediately that rural environments often exacerbate the problem of violence within families in circumstances where gendered assumptions within the law often regard violence in families as 'non-criminal'. In other words, the problem of family violence may not be fully recognised as such because of the way it is conceptualised and defined. Such violence is less recognised, particularly where the so-called private nature of family life makes it more difficult to identify the kind of ongoing threats of violence often experienced by women and children. This is reinforced by the patriarchal nature of rural communities, lack of confidentiality, the anonymity of violence, a lack of services and isolation. Research shows that in circumstances like those faced by small rural towns, it may be difficult to escape or avoid a perpetrator, who might seek the same support and legal services. Rural social supports often protect male offenders (Bourke, 2001: 96). Such situations are often regarded as atypical of the image of rural Australia. On the other hand, violence in Indigenous

Australian communities is usually highly systemic and often relates to long-standing family and community dislocations that can be linked to dispossession. In addition, tensions between Aboriginal people and police and legal authorities are usually connected with Aborigines' treatment in the criminal justice system and their high rates of victimisation.

It is important to emphasise again that violence in rural areas is not simply a matter between perpetrator and victim. It continues because of the structures, cultures and contexts of rural communities. Lisa Bourke (2001) provides examples of these structures that are revealed in research: police may be 'mates' with perpetrators; victims are rarely able to be anonymous when reporting violence; people in powerful positions make claims that 'that sort of thing doesn't happen around here'. They also cite the cultural insensitivity of the criminal justice system towards Indigenous Australians. But the rural context is recognised as a fundamental condition for much of the violence. While the five highest rates of Apprehended Violence Orders (AVOs) were recorded in rural local government areas in New South Wales, rural violence has historically and culturally been constructed as a non-issue. From a governmentality perspective, the definition and calculation of violence needs to be recalibrated in order for government to manage the problem effectively. Reconstructing 'what is violence' remains an important challenge for rural communities, and victims themselves can contribute to broadening the definition and expanding an understanding of the problem (see Kesby, 2005). In the meantime, issues like rural poverty, isolation, lack of educational provision and rural economic restructuring continue to be basic problems underlying strong levels of official and 'unofficial' violence in rural families.

DISCURSIVE REGIMES AND RISK MANAGEMENT IN FAMILIES

Many of these points about the structural antecedents of violence in rural communities are demonstrated in David Thorpe's (1994) study of social work in rural Western Australia. Thorpe accentuates the construction and defining of a problem (and hence how it is to be managed) in the way that the problem is formed through language and concepts—what we could call its discursive formation. The particular form of family violence is defined as 'child abuse'—clearly a serious example of violence in rural communities that is largely hidden in the family. Case records showed intensive inquiries into the behaviours of a very large number of parents, with only a very small proportion resulting in children being assessed as 'at risk'. According to Thorpe, it was the vocabulary around child abuse that led professionals to 'spectacularly miss the point' about the contexts in which allegations arise—that is, the massive over-representation of poor and disadvantaged people, especially single female parent families and Aboriginal people. It showed that the construction of the problem of violence using the term 'child abuse' encouraged a pathologising and blaming of parents, while the actual conditions of these children failed to improve as a consequence of the interventions. Indeed, the signifier of 'abuse' in fact leads parents to be seen as a threat to their children (Thorpe, 1994: 196–9).

However, evidence of social processes that criminalise children, particularly girls and Aborigines, is equally well recorded. Kerry Carrington's (1993) remarkable study in the 1980s shows that girls appearing in court on welfare matters were more likely to receive a custodial sentence than those appearing on criminal offences. The pattern of sentencing was the outcome of the logic of 'preventative intervention' rather than 'pure' judicial logic. 'Deficit discourses' were used to identify 'pre-delinquency', and this classification was deemed sufficient to justify the committal of welfare cases to insti-tutions. Reports presented in courts show the use of a range of deficit discourses—moral, psychological, social—in coming to an assessment about individual girls studied in the survey. They then had practical effects on the way children were chosen, placed and punished by juvenile justice and child welfare authorities alike (1993: 127). A complex web of modern governmental technologies, prima-rily designed to save children from 'bad families', produced what Carrington describes as a highly selective 'delinquency manufactur-ing process' (1993: 1). These findings have recently been substanti-ated in New Zealand research on the life trajectories of women in jail, whose chances as children of escaping a well-worn 'welfare' pathway to incarceration were irrevocably damaged by assump-tions about normal childhood and family held by those authorities charged with acting in support of their 'rights' and 'best interests' (Lashlie, 2010).

In summary, how we construct problems in rural communi-ties has repercussions for how we then go about addressing these problems. For example, criminalising violence in the home draws particular attention to perpetrators and victims, but may miss the importance of the systemic nature of the problem. If one of the main underlying issues with violence is rural poverty brought about by agricultural and economic restructuring or policy changes, a focus only on individual responses and solutions will be misplaced. If poor education provision due to rural isolation leads to a lack of employment opportunities and health problems, the central issue of rural resources needs to be addressed. Also, social problems rarely exist in isolation, and many individuals—such as Indigenous people—have multiple, interrelated issues that will be addressed only through a longer-term perspective on the effects of changing social environments on lifestyles. Bourke (2001) points out that strong traditional understandings of gender, masculinity, sexuality and family lead to an acceptance of violence as a 'natural' response. She argues:

> The need for the acceptance of difference in rural communities, in order that masculinity, sexuality and family may be expressed in various forms beyond existing rigid structures, is clear. It is only through critical analysis of our understanding of these issues in a broader context that social problems in rural areas will really be addressed. (2001: 102)

GOVERNMENTALITY AND FAMILY VIOLENCE

We can see from the example above, which shows how violence in rural families may be defined as non-criminal and hence a non-problem, that defining a problem is a crucial element of the governmentality perspective. A problem comes to be 'known' in particular ways in order for it to be properly managed. In the case of violence against children, knowledge of the child is largely derived from the administrative requirements of the agencies charged with actually managing the protection of children. We can use the governmentality perspective to understand how this way of defining the problem has implications for managing the problem of violence against children. Under mandatory reporting laws, these agencies can include social workers, teachers, police, medical practitioners, neighbours, and so on. So, while there is evidence that the definitions and language of family violence change over time, there is also evidence that changes in governing and management practices shift the gaze on to children and families, and alter how people get counted. That is, there is a level of contingency in the discursive production of the problem child, and there is evidence that an administration's demand to 'know in order to protect' has produced massive surges in the numbers of children 'known to the agency' (McCallum, 2009). Strategies of risk management result in higher rates of reported cases of various kinds of child abuse among disadvantaged groups, which is particularly significant for Aboriginal children. Also, a number of different kinds of events can be reported and counted in the category of child abuse, adding a level of contingency in the calculation of the problem.

The actual term 'child abuse' is quite recent, originating from doctors' knowledge of children with broken bones and other serious injuries encountered in hospital settings during the 1960s, in the same period Colorado paediatricians under C. Henry Kempe invented the 'battered baby syndrome' (McCallum, 2009). Later, in its classification by statistical authorities, the phenomenon of child abuse was rendered into categories of individual actions: 'physical abuse', 'sexual abuse', 'neglect' and 'emotional abuse' (AIHW, 2010a). These actions can be interpreted as perpetrations. They involve illegal acts committed against children for which any reasonable person could have nothing but abhorrence. These categorisations need to be situated within the milieu of poverty and dislocation. The representation of the problem can help to 'spectacularly miss the point', as Thorpe (1994) suggests, about the context of problems. The statistics presented in this way also produce categories within which people might be thought and might think about themselves. The latter is clearly in evidence from personal accounts of the moralising and shaming effects of the federal government's Northern Territory intervention on Aboriginal people accused of child abuse (see Nimmo & Zubrycki, 2008).

CASE STUDY

Imagine you are a social worker in the Northern Territory who travels regularly to a homelands community that is functioning well on many levels but does confront issues around child safety. As a community, the Aboriginal women have decided that the best way to protect children is to set up a child safety service where a group of women patrols the community after dark. (Descriptions of some of these night patrols are incorporated in the *Little Children Are Sacred* report (Wild & Anderson, 2007)). The women's goal is to protect the children, to develop trusting relationships with the children and to encourage the children to go home at night. Your role is to facilitate a meeting with these women every time you visit the community. You are keen to support their work, and provide feedback to your agency about the kinds of supports the community and the women need to address violence and child safety issues. This program is proving effective and yet the changes to community development employment programs are likely to mean that these women will not be paid for their work (Carney, 2007).

Reflective question

• What kind of action would you plan to take? How might the 'governmentality' framework outlined in this chapter assist you to argue the women's case back in your agency and with policy-makers?

This example draws attention to the important functions of governing, and also shows what we can learn from the 'mentalities of government' perspective, including its effects on how people are thought about and think of themselves, or their subjectivity. The *Little Children Are Sacred* report (Wild & Anderson, 2007) highlights the structures influencing rural and remote communities and their responses to stress, isolation and poverty.

More recently, however, research has tended to highlight the diversity of these communities, as well as the range of responses people have to rural problems. This diversity is demonstrated in the different and varied ways in which people involved in family violence *experience* those structures; for example, that gender relations are not transmitted in an unmediated way, but are open to various interpretations and therefore capable of modification and change. Gender and patriarchy can be seen as structured top-down suppression and oppression, but also as a point of convergence among culturally and historically specific sets of relations. In Sarah Wendt's (2009) study in the Barossa Valley, for example, local cultures provided frameworks for women to understand their experiences of violence and respond to it, within the frameworks of understanding of those cultures. The meanings given to self-reliance, community pride, privacy, family inheritance, marriage and religion all impacted on the ways in which women made sense of situations, and sought to find solutions. Very often, the strength of these cultures meant that women were encouraged to cope on their own, to keep silent about domestic violence, and to understand how institutions like property, marriage and religion can be more powerful and influential than the women themselves. But they also provided a space, in participation with others, including human service workers, for discourses about the rural to be unravelled and analysed in order to enable alternative pathways to be imagined and found (Wendt, 2009: 154–6).

POLICY AND PRACTICE

In the policy discussion preceding the Victorian *Children, Youth and Families Act* 2005, the goal of the new Act was to reflect international trends in responding to the needs of children and families. Child services policy in Victoria set a direction that was seen as a model for other states and territories in how to respond to the increased rates of notifications and substantiations of child abuse that have been seen over the past decade. Australia, the United Kingdom and North America had earlier adopted a 'regulatory' child protection orientation to child abuse, as distinct from the family service orientation long practised in countries like Sweden, Germany, Belgium and the Netherlands. In the lead-up to the new Act, policy analysts claimed that the family services approach provided easier access to a wider range of services and assistance than regulatory systems (VDHS, 2003: vii). 'Family service systems' placed more emphasis on working voluntarily with parents over longer periods, compared with the earlier, more coercive approach. A regulatory approach worked well when responding to episodes of significant harm but was less effective in dealing with more chronic cases of ongoing neglect. Recent approaches to reform have stressed the importance of a spectrum of responses to families' needs, while retaining the capacity to apply 'tough sanctions'. Mandated agencies need to work in partnership with other agencies, and these partnerships work best when the people who are engaged with these services see the services as procedurally fair and as treating families and all concerned with respect. Liberal notions of self-government flavoured the approach:

> child protection regulation should build on, or interact more with, parents' own 'private regulation', or self-regulation. Government regulation should respond to how effectively private regulation is working *and can be encouraged to work better.* (VDHS, 2003: viii, emphasis in original)

In 2003, a government-ordered review claimed that if the current administrative arrangements for child protection were maintained, one in five children in the cohort born in Victoria in 2003 would be notified for suspected child abuse or neglect during their childhood or adolescence; child protection could no longer be an 'emergency service' (VDHS, 2003: vi). So the virtues of the new order would in large part be based on the necessity for changing the child abuse notification and substantiation processes. There would be more preventative and diversionary strategies, less resort to statutory and court processes, and a greater opportunity for children to become part of a family by acting earlier to provide permanent care. This was to be achieved through building 'community-partnerships', and encouraging vulnerable families to access support by providing more responsive and flexible services. These strategies would be supported by an expanded 'community infrastructure'. In the VDHS (2003) *Final Report of the Child Protection Outcomes Project*, community infrastructure is described as Community Child and Family Support Centres in local areas, locally coordinated 'community-based' services including 'child protection, family support, health, police and schools, and the development of intermediate level responses that allow for dialogue and deliberation with families outside of formal legal processes' (VDHS, 2003: xiv). Exposing the seasonality of the term 'community', community-based solutions to family governance would now entail a gaze onto whole populations in order to assess family needs (Bauman, 2000).

Here, the reformist aspirations for protecting children were unmistakable. Child protection cases would be managed in the community, and decisions about either reunification or out-of-home care would be sped up. What does it mean that child protection or police are now understood as 'community'? In terms of formal legal process, DHS would be required to explain to the Children's Court why it would *not* be in the best interests of a child or young person to work towards a longer-term out-of-home care arrangement. There has been a similar reversal of the onus of proof in New South Wales. In addition, managing cases in the community was to be achieved through voluntary child-care agreements to place children in out-of-home care, a provision in the legislation that was borrowed from the *Community Services Act* 1970, which was amalgamated into the new 2005 Act. These written agreements between a parent and a service provider must take into account the wishes of the child, and the parties may agree to one or more extensions for a period not exceeding six months. In the case of long-term child-care agreements, the period may not exceed two years. Agreements may be terminated by any party giving notice in writing. Under the previous *Children and Young Persons Act* 1989 guidelines, a precondition for making a permanent care order was that the child's parent had not had care of the child for a period of at least two years.

From the description of community engagement outlined in the policy documents cited above, there is a need to exercise care about how to interpret policy directions that uncritically propose community participation as the magic bullet for problems of empowering people. As many authors have suggested, following the publication of *Participation: The new tyranny?* (Cooke & Kothari, 2001),

> the effects of power are not intrinsically stable; they appear to be so only if the knowledges and practices constituting prevailing inequalities continue to be reproduced. But it is not just elites who undertake this work; simply acting out socially defined roles and identities implicates dominated subjects in the transmission and reproduction of the very discourses and practices that constitute them as inferior. Indeed, power is most effective and most insidious where it is normalized, where self-expectation, self-regulation, and self-discipline generate compliant subjects who actively reproduce hegemonic assemblages of power without being 'forced' to do so. (Kesby, 2005: 2040)

Community participation can be mobilised to serve a wide variety of political agendas, and participatory approaches can impose, not overcome, power relations when delivered as a 'technocratic cargo' (Kesby, 2005: 2037). Indeed, as we can observe in our descriptions of rural cultures, practitioners often erroneously imagine local communities as discrete and socially homogeneous. In a discussion of his research in the highly politically charged context of Zimbabwe, Mike Kesby reaffirms the importance of understanding and engaging with power, rather than merely avoiding it. Community participatory discourses can be revalorised and retheorised using the theoretical standpoint of 'mentalities of governing', and are especially effective when community participation is used to outmanoeuvre dominant forms of power. Community participation needs to be able to reframe the assumptions that structure rural cultures in ways that enable the context of family violence to be acknowledged, named and transcended.

CONCLUSION

This chapter has reviewed different sites of family violence in rural settings in an effort to understand how the governmentality literature can assist in analysing the forms of power at stake in these relations and how these power relations can be changed. The shaping and defining of social problems becomes critical to how these problems are managed. The aim is to convey the levels of contingency in accounting for problem families and children, including children who are vulnerable to criminalisation and possible imprisonment. There is evidence that expanded definitions of violence and abuse can bring to light previously hidden forms of violence in the domestic scene, and bring about a broader understanding of abusive behaviours and conditions. There is equally good evidence that changes in intervention and management practices can assist families and individuals to address violence in the home. In addition, welfare administrations produce categories in which people might be thought of and might think about themselves. Expanding a shared knowledge of the subjective and experiential aspects of violence is an important means of confronting violence in rural settings. Sharing this knowledge and its underlying assumptions provides opportunities for citizens in rural environments to participate in processes that undermine the antecedents of violent behaviours.

RECOMMENDED READING

Bauman, Z. (2000) *Community: Seeking safety in an insecure world*. Polity Press, Cambridge.

Carney, M. (2007) Tracking the intervention (videorecording). *Four Corners*, ABC TV, 5 November.

Cashmore, J. (2001) Child protection in the new millennium. *Social Policy Research Centre Newsletter*, 79, 1–5.

Concerned Australians (2010) *This is What We Said: Australian Aboriginal people give their views on the Northern Territory Intervention*. Vega Press, Melbourne.

Hacking, I. (1991) The making and moulding of child abuse. *Critical Inquiry*, 17, 257–88.

Lashlie, C. (2010) *The Power of Mothers*. HarperCollins, Auckland.

Parton, N. (1991) *Governing the Family. Child care, child protection and the state*. Macmillan, Basingstoke.

Tedmanson, D. & Wadiwel, D. (2010) Neoptolemus: The governmentality of new race/pleasure wars? *Culture and Organization*, 16(1), 7–22.

10

INTEGRATING MIGRANTS AND REFUGEES IN RURAL SETTINGS

Linda Briskman

Seven hundred rolls did the baker bake today.
Seven hundred guests did the town receive today.[1]

CHAPTER OBJECTIVES

- To outline a brief history and discuss the context of migrant and refugee settlement in Australia.
- To identify factors that both enhance and inhibit migrant resettlement.
- To discuss theoretical constructs and discourses related to welcoming diverse populations.
- To consider the approach rural practitioners might take in their work with people who are refugees.

INTRODUCTION

In 1999 I wrote somewhat harshly (Briskman, 1999) of what I saw then as the deep conservatism of rural communities, places shrouded in monoculturalism that contrasted with the groundswell of diversity of urban settings. I spoke of the perception of rural

---

[1] Extract from a song written by Kavisha Mazella and Arnold Zable, which describes the kind deeds of the townsfolk of the small island of Zakynthos in the Ionian Sea. It was performed at The Boîte in Melbourne in 2003.

residents as being the keepers of traditional beliefs and values, and often receiving labels such as redneck, anti-diversity and even racist. Although this perception was perhaps part of the myth-making associated with the rural milieu, particularly as it did not acknowledge successes in migrant settlement, it was less contestable when it came to refugees. Although migrants have settled in rural Australia over a long period of time, talk of refugees and even less of asylum seekers had barely permeated Australian cities and was certainly not in the rural lexicon.

This chapter explores social work practice with migrant and refugee communities in rural Australia. It examines the ways in which rural communities have responded, highlights some of the debates and then contemplates—including through a case study and reflective questions—how a social worker may navigate through this area of practice.

My interest in the area of migration does not stem from immersion in practice in this arena when I worked in rural Victoria as a social worker throughout the 1980s. Although in the course of my work I came across migrant communities, there were few that had encounters with my own professional social work practice. My interest emerged at a time when a steady flow of asylum seekers began reaching Australian shores from 1999, and were subject to the harsh policy of mandatory detention. In the years since, I have watched many of those who were eventually released from immigration detention on the Temporary Protection Visa (TPV) policy that was in place from 1999 until 2008 settle in rural areas. At the same time, a planned settlement process for refugees under the humanitarian program (explained in the next section) took place.

I observed during the harshest years of mandatory detention policies that much support for refugees and asylum seekers came from rural areas, particularly the formation in 2001 of the organisation Rural Australians for Refugees (RAR). RAR drew together rural people from throughout Australia who were affronted by the government's asylum seeker and refugee policies. As well as offering direct support to asylum seekers, the overall aim of RAR was to turn around public opinion; thus its intent was highly political as well as humanitarian (Coombs, 2005). During these years, there was little formal opportunity for social workers and other service providers to alleviate the distress, as the services accorded to other refugees were not granted to those on TPVs. Nonetheless, informal supports emerged—including from church and community groups, many of which showed great compassion for the refugees. Many employers embraced the new pool of labour and, through work-force participation in country towns, acceptance of people from Middle Eastern countries in particular grew. Social movements and labour movements hence contributed to a turning point for the rural milieu.

In late 2008 I returned to the rural community where I had prac-tised as a social worker and was amazed at the transformation of this town into what is now a refugee-welcoming community where men, women and children from far-flung lands are part of the dynamic community fabric. Nonetheless, as will be argued in this chapter, there is no room for complacency, as settlement processes can be fraught, and social workers need to be mindful of policies, debates, theoretical drivers and practice approaches to overcome structural barriers.

MIGRANTS AND REFUGEES IN REGIONAL AND RURAL AREAS

Although there have been specific programs that have led to people from other countries moving to regional and rural areas, this chapter does not delve into settlement policy in detail. Instead, it starts from the premise that migrants and refugees have contributed to the social capital of rural areas and, although there have been times when the struggle for social cohesion has been problematic, there are stories of success where the rights of immigrants and refugees have been achieved and where the needs and expectations of the wider commu-nity have been met.

In general, *migrants* freely move to a country in search of better economic or lifestyle opportunities than those experienced in their own country. They are unlikely to be moving for fear of persecu-tion or oppression. Of course, this does not make it a non-stressful event, for all people on the move to a new country face settlement difficulties, which may include problems with cultural adjustment and job-seeking. Those with children have to assist them readjust to a new setting for their education and friendship networks. However, unlike a refugee, a migrant's departure is generally planned with the opportunity to take with them personal items and to farewell loved ones (Briskman & Fiske, 2009: 137). Unlike refu-gees, there is the option to return if they are not satisfied with their move. Migrants generally experience less community suspicion than refugees—especially onshore refugees—as migration is viewed by the populace as an orderly process that does not conflict with Australia's norms and population policy.

Distinctive from the category of immigrant, a *refugee* is a person who has been found by the United Nations High Commission for Refugees (UNHCR), or a delegated authority (such as the Department of Immigration and Citizenship in Australia), to meet the definitions of a refugee contained in the 1951 Refugee Convention. The Convention defines a refugee as a person who is outside her or his country of nationality, and who is unable or unwilling to return to that country due to a well-founded fear of persecution on the basis of one of the following:

- race
- religion
- nationality
- membership of a particular social group, or
- political opinion.

Refugees are known as 'offshore' refugees if their claims are assessed prior to them coming to Australia. An *asylum seeker* is a person who has applied for formal recognition of refugee status and is awaiting an answer. Often an asylum seeker has had similar experiences to a refugee, but has not had access to the protections that come with formal refugee status. If they arrive in Australia without identity documents or a visa, they are described as 'unlawful' (Briskman & Fiske, 2009: 136). Offshore refugees are the most likely to have contact with social workers and other community supports. They have often come from refugee camps, and once in Australia are entitled to a range of support services.

A brief overview of critical policy moments in white settlement in Australia provides an introduction to the prospects and limits of Australia as a receiving country for both immigrants and refugees. Michael Grewcock (2009) aptly explains some of the tensions and contradictions in the welcome of outsiders. Although, as he recounts, the White Australia Policy was abolished in the 1970s—which then allowed permanent migration from non-European sources—there remains a continuation of its ideological underpinnings. Furthermore, although the concept of multiculturalism took hold in Australia at institutional and state levels, these have been contested, with proponents of its demise seeing it as divisive rather than cohesive.

It is important to remember that six million of Australia's residents arrived since 1947, or are the children or grandchildren of migrants. Over the past century, people from 240 countries have come to Australia (MacLeod, 2006). Furthermore, around 98 per cent of the population are either immigrants or descendants of immigrants, and it is only the Indigenous peoples of Australia who can truly be said to have a traditional claim on the land. This fact is often forgotten in debates about who has a rightful place in Australia, a debate that particularly came to the forefront when Pauline Hanson, who formed the One Nation Party, was elected to the federal parliament as the Member for Oxley in 1996. Among her policy planks was opposition to both Indigenous rights and immigration, speaking out against the 'Aboriginal industry' and multiculturalism. In some parts of rural Australia—particularly Queensland—she galvanised support, with populations disaffected by population decline, economic problems and dwindling services seeing her as a hope for their exclusion from mainstream policies of government.

Although the wave of refugees over the last decade has had an impact on rural communities, it builds upon early migrant settlement experiences in those communities. There are many rural areas in Australia that have settled migrants from Western Europe, and they have become an accepted part of rural community life. After World War II, refugees were welcomed into Australia to provide a labour force for the Snowy Mountains scheme in New South Wales. After the end of the Vietnam War, Australia accepted refugees from that country. Some settled in rural areas, with mixed success at a time when service providers and others were less well informed about refugees than they are today.

Although conservatism is increasing in the political realm world-wide (Alston, 2009b: 345), over the last decade there has been a rural revolution in terms of both attitudes and settlement numbers. Rural Australia is now home to refugees from various countries, and with different skills and experiences and various modes of arriving, building on the contribution of waves of migrants before them. However, even though migrants and refugees in rural areas are gaining increasing acceptance, when asked to consider the proposition that 'accepting immigrants from different countries makes Australia stronger', people have responded differently. The replies reveal that residents of capital cities are more likely to be in agreement than those living in regional centres and rural areas (Markus et al., 2009: 135).

Since the mid-1990s the Department of Immigration has fostered a steady stream of migrants to provincial centres (Carrington & Marshall, 2008: 117). An increase from 2004 was intended to create a more balanced dispersal of migrants across Australia and help prevent a 'cultural chasm' opening up between the country and capital cities. It was hoped that such dispersal would create a flow-on effect, and that future arrivals would follow the lead of others. It was also believed that migrants would find early employment and therefore experience more rapid integration into the host communities. (The broader question of rural employment, discussed in Chapter 6, should be considered alongside this chapter.) In its 2008–09 annual report the department states that it continues to support an increase in humanitarian settlement in regional areas in order to achieve a more 'balanced distribution of refugees'. Other recent policy statements speak of developing a long-term strategy for increased settlement in rural and regional locations.

There is an underlying premise that refugees in the humanitarian stream would help meet demands for less-skilled labour needed in rural economies (Carrington & Marshall, 2008: 117). This last premise is among the most controversial for, as Jon Stratton (2009) points out, in the Howard years of government (1996–2007), when Australia increased its migration program for skilled labour in the guise of the 457 visa,[2] this was in fact employer driven. He notes that 'the visa typifies the neoliberal understanding of the primacy of the market', and furthermore raises concerns that 'boatpeople' have not only been racialised but also 'classed' in the way they have been constructed as unskilled, which is in fact little more than a persuasive myth.

WHAT CREATES SUCCESS?

There is an increasing body of literature and reports referring to the success factors and inhibitors relating to migrant and refugee settlement patterns in rural areas, and social workers can explore these—including in relation to their own practice settings. There are some broad leads that can assist such an analysis. In migrant resettlement, there are success stories and problems—for example, research has revealed that new settlers were easily absorbed into the

---

[2] Information on this visa is readily available from the Department of Immigration and Citizenship website at <www.immi.gov.au>.

Victorian locality of Shepparton, while Toowoomba in Queensland struggled. Using a social capital framework (elaborated upon in Chapter 2), Kerry Carrington and Neil Marshall (2008: 118) argue that Shepparton had developed extensive networks of bridging social capital, which facilitated the integration of new arrivals. On the other hand, Toowomba possessed strong reserves of bonding social capital among residents but little in the way of bridging social capital. Employment is a major factor in the welcoming of refugees. In its program of regional settlement, the Immigration Department has chosen centres with this in mind, together with such factors as housing and service availability and a welcoming environment (Carrington & Marshall, 2008: 117).

A literature review prepared by the Refugee Council of Australia (RCOA) (2010) reveals that the refugees and humanitarian migrants who have settled in Australia since Federation have had a profound impact on enhancing the nation's social, cultural and economic life. Although the contribution of Australia to hosting the settlement of refugees is the primary focus, there is no doubt that refugees make substantial contributions to their new country—expanding consumer markets for local goods, opening new markets, bringing in new skills, creating employment and filling empty employment niches. Australia's refugees and humanitarian entrants have found success in every field of endeavour, including the arts, sport, media, science, research, business, and civic and community life. The positive impact of refugees has especially been felt in regional and rural Australia. In recent times, rural areas have experienced large-scale departures of people, resulting in skills losses, lack of local entrepreneurship, business closures and the loss of social capital and services. The young age profile of humanitarian entrants makes a very positive contribution to the rural labour market.

The RCOA study also reveals some barriers encountered by refugees, especially those who have not had the opportunity to attain qualifications and employment experience because of the nature of their migration experience. Those who have spent protracted periods in refugee camps or immigration detention are likely to be affected, as are many women arriving under the humanitarian program. A lack of Australian work experience can present problems, as many employers do not recognise overseas work experience. Refugees may struggle to get the entry-level jobs that enable them to gain experience.

When the Australian Council of Heads of Schools of Social Work (ACHSSW) conducted the People's Inquiry into Detention (described in the case study following), rural successes were conveyed. These included a union organiser in a New South Wales rural town who contested the views of the far right political party Australia First (which campaigned against refugees working in industry), stating that the Afghan workers in the meat industry had a good reputation and benefited Australian industry. Similarly, citrus growers in another rural area said that there was a desperate labour need and that people from other countries were loyal and hard workers. The inquiry also heard of refugees who had established successful businesses in rural areas (Briskman et al., 2008).

CONTESTED GROUND

Despite the success stories, social workers should not ignore the variations in attitudes and experiences of resettlement. According to the review by the RCOA, studies have shown that discrimination exists in employment, including racist comments in work environments. Discrimination can be triggered by language ability, accent, name, appearance, gender or religious customs.

The media are where many people—including social workers—gain information about migrants and refugees. It is in the area of asylum seekers that the greatest media impact has been felt, as there is unwarranted hysteria directed at the arrival of boats in Australia, even though the numbers of people involved are relatively small. Some sections of the media avoid good news stories and pay scant attention to the successful movement of refugees to rural areas. There is a barrier to social cohesion when the publicity is negative—for example, as Suvendrini Perera (2007) depicts in relation to the Sudanese in Tamworth in New South Wales. Here Sudanese refugees were positioned as unfit subjects for citizenship and as a threat to 'our way of life', with one councillor voting to exclude the Sudanese (Perera, 2007: 9). Chapter 5 discusses the stigma that can be associated with mental health in rural areas; through populist sentiment and media hyperbole, similar forms of stigma can apply to refugees.

As the newest residents, refugees may not be at the forefront of the concerns of rural communities. They may have to situate themselves where diversity is not always valued and where Aboriginal peoples have been denigrated and denounced. Given this context, it is hardly surprising that reaching out to migrants is often tenuous, and it is 'visible' migrant groups that often bear the brunt of racism. In Australia in recent times, we have seen attacks on Indian students as well as the portrayal of other groups as perpetrators of crime. The headcovering worn by some Muslim women has encountered strong critiques, including labelling of the practice as 'un-Australian', with the underlying proposition that Western 'freedoms' should be imposed on others.

Some rural communities struggle against a belief that they are second-class citizens, and try to exercise their right to adequate funding and recognition. In times of the downfall of the primary industry sector, there may be less reaching out to the newly arrived as labour force needs are not paramount. Rural areas have been affected by the dominance of neo-liberal policies and the privatisation of services. Such policy drivers have caused a decline in collectivism and led to a general apathy towards those in disadvantaged situations (Alston, 2009b: 345).

In addition, some rural communities—particularly those with a limited fiscal base—may lack economic resilience or human capital. For example, the diminishment of government service provision creates more reliance on the non-government sector and volunteers, and these resources are finite. Given that community attitudes to refugees may be tenuous, they may not be given priority over other sectors of the community in both service delivery and volunteer effort.

Service tensions arise for the newly arrived. Rural areas frequently lament the lack of available social work services, and the increase in population may not be met with an increase in service provision. There may also be a lack of emphasis on the particular needs of those who require specialised assistance. An emphasis on fast throughput in the delivery of services in some cases does not bode well for traumatised refugees who have needs over and above the general population, underpinned by both cultural factors and traumatising experiences.

WELCOMING REFUGEES: THEORETICAL INSIGHTS

Given the difficulties outlined above, how can social workers contribute to fostering social change? The song lyrics at the start of this chapter depict the welcoming of a small Greek island community when the townsfolk greeted a boat of strangers. Recently, news spread that, in response to its shrinking population, the mayor of the Italian village of Riace in Italy invited refugees to settle there. In Australia, and out of concern for asylum seekers, there have been reports that the Torres Strait Islander community of Warankuwu has asked the federal government to send refugees there. How common are these positive stories that reach the news, and what has the response been in rural Australia? By drawing on such potential for welcome, social workers are in a good position to muster community strengths.

A critical social work perspective allows social workers to reflect upon how dominant ideologies shape people's lives, and opens the way for a discussion of what methods social workers can adopt in their practice with these populations. The theoretical examples below provide introductory leads for examining how theory and practice meld together in a rural setting; social workers can then draw on other relevant constructs that apply to the context in which they work. Most importantly, by reflecting on our work through our rich knowledge base and practice wisdom, we can keep to the forefront the impact of subjugation, oppression, racism and structural disadvantage (Briskman et al., 2009: 9).

A *human rights* approach can go some way towards ensuring that the rights of both asylum seekers and rural communities are prioritised. Human rights constructs from a social work perspective are for the most vulnerable, and it can be argued that it is refugees who fall into this category. However, it is important to recognise that human rights are for all and, for a social worker to be effective, the needs of all rural constituents need to be taken into account. When rights appear to compete, a process of respectful dialogue is the best way of tackling the tensions.

Consistent with human rights frameworks, an understanding by social workers of *constructs of whiteness* contributes to an awareness of how the 'othering' of specific groups may result in their exclusion from full participation in rural society. One of the key problems here is that 'whiteness' is invisible, and thus remains unrecognised and is rarely discussed. As Aileen Moreton-Robinson (2000) says in relation to Indigenous people, 'whiteness remains the invisible omnipresent norm' (2000: xix). If we contemplate the impact of these factors, we should not be resistant to confronting the racism that can arise from discarding human rights or not recognising the 'whiteness' imperative.

Although it can cause discomfort for many—including social workers employed by mainstream organisations—recognition of how *racism* can occur at various levels is a starting point for engaging in culturally sensitive practice with refugees and migrants. Racism is not just about violent acts and overt racial slurs. It can unwittingly be included in policy documentation and practice tenets, so engaging in critical reflection on practices that directly affect social work practice is essential in challenging this issue. By integrating *anti-oppressive and anti-racist* theorising in approaches to practice, there is increased scope for recognition of the issues and for finding ways to resolve them.

Although it cannot be said that *social capital theory* falls within the critical genre, it is important to contemplate as it has been influential in helping us to understand the lens through which rural stakeholders may view a migration flow. Drawing on emerging social capital theory enables social workers to put themselves in the shoes of dominant rural groups while analysing the question of benefit to both the migrant and the refugee. Robert Putnam's view of social capital as comprising networks of civil engagement is drawn on by Carrington and Marshall (2008: 118) as an explanatory tool that increasingly is being used in multicultural issues. For Carrington and Marshall (2008: 119), for social capital to evolve productively in regional centres there are three elements to be considered. These may be useful for social workers in their practice, including advocacy for policy change:

1 *bonding social capital* that focuses inwards, reinforcing accepted mores and identity within particular groups
2 *bridging social capital* that is directed outwards and encourages linkages and communication between disparate groups within a community, and
3 *governmental social capital*, which refers to the competence of organisational structures to work with and complement community frameworks of interaction.

THE ROLE OF SOCIAL WORKERS

Uschi Bay (2009: 280) points to the importance of adopting an anti-oppressive and empowerment approach to working in rural and remote communities. For Bay, critical social workers must engage with the socio-political dimensions of interlocking patterns of power and influence at the personal, cultural and structural levels. Alston (2009b) alerts us to the political difficulties:

> In recent decades, much of the Western world has experienced a move towards more conservative politics, a political shift paralleled by a move towards a more conservative society in general. (2009b: 345)

Increasingly, social workers have contact with asylum seekers and refugees, and recognise them as a group that struggles for acceptance (Nipperess & Briskman, 2009: 66). By keeping a human rights perspective to the forefront, we have a framework for analysing whether we are conducting our practice in fair and humane ways. It is important for social workers to understand the struggles that have faced refugees, both abroad and in Australia, in order to devise the most appropriate ways of responding to and supporting them. Social workers must remember that refugees may have experienced torture and trauma in their countries of origin. Furthermore, in the host country of Australia, those who have been detained have lost—often for many years—the right to liberty that most of us enjoy, and long-term detention has had social and emotional impacts. Those who arrive through the humanitarian program frequently struggle to have their economic and social rights realised as they make their way through Australian society and experience community and institutional racism.

Not all migrants and refugees in rural communities have achieved formal citizenship status. Nonetheless, as permanent residents they are entitled to a feeling of belonging in the sense of social rather than legal citizenship. There may be barriers to people from some cultural groups attaining citizenship—particularly the provisions of the citizenship test, which require substantial knowledge of Australian society and a degree of literacy, English language proficiency and confidence in an examination setting. Some people may be embarrassed about what they see as their own limitations. Social workers can help people through these structural barriers, to ensure that they are not excluded from attaining full citizenship rights that people from Western countries may achieve with more ease.

Effective service provision is crucial. In a study examining regional humanitarian settlement in the Victorian town of Ballarat, an integral ingredient for success was 'the people in many of the key service delivery positions who have acquired valuable skills in working with humanitarian entrants' (Piper & Associates, 2009: 54). Acquiring these skills requires a combination of effort by social work educators, rural practitioners and organisations delivering services to rural constituents.

Finally, social workers can take heed of the political work that has gone on in rural areas, particularly the work of Rural Australians for Refugees. Not only was RAR a powerhouse of activity in confronting policy concerns, it contributed to turning around the type of perceptions of rural areas alluded to early in the chapter. The words of one of the founders of RAR, Ann Coombs (2005), should resonate here about the effectiveness of RAR's activities:

> It simply confirmed to me what I already knew—that regional Australia is not the redneck, conservative monolith that most people think. The country has changed. Country people are far more diverse than city dwellers realise. Refugee supporters might still be in the minority in the bush but the fact that RAR groups are thriving from Mt Isa to Cootamundra is an indication that regional Australians can be as passionate about this issue as anyone else.

CASE STUDY: SOCIAL WORK AND RURAL ADVOCACY

In 2005, the Australian Council of Heads of Schools of Social Work (ACHSSW) initiated the People's Inquiry into Detention. For the purposes of this chapter, this case study is important for two reasons. First, it shows how social work can take the lead in advocacy and activism to expose unjust policies and practices. Second, through ensuring that the voices of rural people—refugees, advocates and employers—were included in the process, it revealed first-hand experiences of selected communities.

The People's Inquiry was established by the ACHSSW from deep concern about the mandatory immigration detention of asylum seekers. The purpose of this citizens' inquiry was twofold: to endeavour to influence policy change and to expose the situation of detention, including the harms done to men, women and children. The inquiry team ran public hearings in urban and rural areas, and also received written submissions from people with experience of detention. One-third of those who gave verbal testimony had been incarcerated in detention centres.

The example below was presented to the inquiry by rural advocates, and illustrates the difficulties that refugees face and the need for social work awareness and support.

> Some call the TPV 'detention without the wire'. They become more pessimistic about ever obtaining a permanent visa and family reunion. The refugees' wives cannot understand why it is taking so long to bring them here and that is another level

of stress for the men. Separations of five to six years are very damaging to marriages and children, some of whom have never met their fathers. The men work seven days a week to dull the psychological pain. They have done this for over five years and are now exhausted and breaking down. We know of none who aren't suffering from stress, poor sleep, night-mares, anxiety and depression. (Cited in Briskman et al., 2008: 343)

Exercise 1

Ali is a refugee from a war-torn country who has settled in a rural area with a population of 10 000. He presents himself at the local Centrelink office and is referred to a social worker as he appears depressed and alienated. The social worker quickly identifies some of the major difficulties he is encountering, including the delay in reunification with his family, who are in a refugee camp abroad; Ali's difficulty in obtaining employment; being the subject of racist taunts from time to time; and feeling isolated, bored and lonely.

As the social worker in the situation:

- What skills and knowledge can help you provide a sound service for Ali?
- What theories can guide the way you enact your social work practice in this instance?
- How will you prioritise Ali's needs?
- What strategies will you put in place?

Exercise 2

Danu, age ten, has arrived in a small rural town of fewer than 3000 people, where her parents have taken up professional roles as skilled migrants. Danu is left to her own devices for long periods of time, including caring for her seven-year-old brother. She is referred to you by the school as she often appears listless and has few friends. Although her English is not well developed, she conveys to you that she misses her home-land and especially her large extended family. She is having difficulty coping with the style of learning in school and does not feel that the other students wish to befriend her.

In your social work role:

- How would you conceptualise the issues facing Danu?
- What role would you take with the school and family to resolve her distress?
- How would you familiarise yourself with policies that relate to the support services that are in place for children of skilled migrants?
- Are there community supports that could be put in place for Danu?

SUMMARY

This chapter has presented an overview of issues of settlement of migrants, and more specifically refugees. In providing an outline of prospects and barriers, it calls on social workers to utilise their theoretical and practice knowledge base and to contemplate robust advocacy in striving for acceptance of diversity and the well-being of newly arrived groups in rural communities.

RECOMMENDED READING

Kenny, M. & Fiske, L. (2009) Social work practice with refugees and asylum seekers. In *In the Shadow of the Law: The legal context of social work practice*. Federation Press, Sydney.

Martin, J. (2006) Social work with refugees and asylum seekers. In W.H. Chui and J. Wilson (eds), *Social Work and Human Services Best Practice*. Federation Press, Sydney.

11

GOVERNING HOMELANDS IN DESERT AUSTRALIA

Uschi Bay

My name is Dr Gawirrin Gumana AO of Gangan, and I am one of the old people who fought for our Land Rights. Government, I would like to pass this on to you, my words now.

If you are looking for people to move out, if you want to move us around like cattle, like others who have already gone to the cities and towns, I tell you, I don't want to play these games.

Government, if you don't help our Homelands, and try to starve me from my land, I tell you, you can kill me first. You will have to shoot me. Listen to me.—Social Justice Report submission, 2009

CHAPTER OBJECTIVES

- To identify the debates about the viability of remote Aboriginal settlements.
- To describe different kinds of remote desert settlements and livelihoods.
- To explore service delivery models for remote desert settlements.
- To discuss the Northern Territory intervention and claims of child sexual abuse and neglect.
- To draw on anti-racist social work theory to guide practice.

INTRODUCTION

My introduction to the complex, challenging and pressing issues confronting desert settlements was through the 'desert knowledge movement' in Australia. A Desert Knowledge Cooperative Research

Centre (DKCRC) was funded by the Commonwealth government from 2003 to 2010, and it brought together Aboriginal and non-Aboriginal researchers from various disciplines around the nation, and included Aboriginal elders, local settlement residents, town leaders and livestock graziers to engage in developing sustainable desert livelihood opportunities. For me, this experience highlighted the many political issues involved in attempting to characterise desert settlements. The research process highlighted the contests that exist over knowledge, land, power and identity. Post-structuralist theorists indicate that these are crucial concepts, with major effects on who can access resources and whose rights are recognised and enacted. In this chapter, I explore the debates about service delivery viability, and discuss methods for engaging with remote desert settlements, advocating particularly for adequate and appropriate services to homelands resettled by Aboriginal people.

I will draw on the recent Northern Territory Inquiry into the Child Protections System (2010) to illustrate the challenges for desert dwellers who often 'have only a distant, marginal voice in political and policy decision making' (Davies & Holcombe, 2009: 363). Major changes were introduced recently to Aboriginal livelihoods through the Northern Territory Intervention, including compulsory income management, changes to the Community Development Employment Project (CDEP)—a primary source of income for Aboriginal people living and working in remote communities—and the compulsory acquisition of Aboriginal townships through five-year leases. These changes were introduced without any consultation with the Aboriginal peoples affected by these policies, even as these changes meant a major shock to sustainable livelihood strategies for Aboriginal people in desert Australia. Through the new 'Working Future' initiative, the Northern Territory government is 'now seeking to urbanize those remaining Indigenous peoples living in remote communities, by moving financial support away from outstations to twenty larger Aboriginal communities it calls "Territory Growth Towns"' (Short, 2010: 60).

Leading social work authors using an anti-oppressive and empowerment perspective have developed strong anti-racist theory that adds much to social work practice (Dominelli, 2008; Briskman, 2007). Both Lena Dominelli and Linda Briskman promote critical reflexivity and political action by social workers in relation to institutional racism. There is strong evidence of major underfunding and lack of adequate service provision to homeland communities in desert Australia (Briskman, 2007). The challenge for social workers is to work out how to contribute effectively to the community development programs and early intervention services in rural and remote desert Australia within the historical context of much systems failure.

DESCRIBING DESERT AUSTRALIA

The Australian desert region covers two-thirds of the landmass of the continent, and spans five states and one territory (Young & Guenther, 2008: 177). Most Australians live in coastal cities or regional towns, and Australia's desert region is sparsely populated—only about 3 per cent of the Australian population lives there, and about half of those people live in five regional service and mining centres. In characterising desert settlements, Desert Knowledge Cooperative researchers aimed to take into account the population size and composition, as well as the socio-economic aspects, of these settlements as a basis for further research. A few key observations will contextualise the following discussion about some of the issues facing remote Aboriginal settlements in desert Australia.

There are five larger settlements in desert Australia, each with between 18 000 and 49 999 residents. These are Alice Springs, Kalgoorlie, Mount Isa, Whyalla and Broken Hill. These settlements have a predominantly non-Aboriginal population. Historically, it is important to understand that Aboriginal people were prohibited from towns in desert Australia. For instance, Alice Springs—located on traditional central Arrernte land known as Mparntwe to local Arrernte people—was gazetted in 1888 and 'Aboriginal people were displaced to the outskirts of town by the development of the pastoral industry' (Satour, 2009). From 1900 to 1964, Alice Springs township was declared a prohibited area to Aboriginal people, who settled on the perimeter of town in what are now called 'town camps'. Aboriginal people in these camps provided a labour force for the railway line, and worked for the non-Aboriginal pastoralists as domestics and farm hands, stockmen and cooks (Satour, 2009). Aboriginal people's labour was vital to Australia's desert cattle industry, and without their work this industry would not have survived. Aboriginal people were 'paid' in rations (flour, sugar and tea), tobacco and some clothing until the 1960s. The pastoral industry put pressure on Aboriginal people's livelihoods because cattle spoilt waterholes, and destroyed grasses and plants—thus depleting bush tucker and game for hunting. The battles over land also resulted in killings and massacres of Aboriginal people—for instance, 'over one hundred Warlpiri men and women and children were shot by police and stockmen in retaliation for the killing of dingo trapper Fred Brooks' in 1928 (Ikuntji artists, 2010).

Aboriginal people were forced off their traditional lands, and this disruption to their livelihood strategies meant that they were made reliant on the ration stations set up by governments or by Lutheran missionaries—for example, at Lake Killalparinna (1866) or Hermannsburg (1877)—for food. The missions further disrupted traditional lifestyles by prohibiting Aboriginal cultural practices. Government assimilation policy in Australia from the late 1950s to 1972 sought to bring all Aboriginal people still living in the bush into missions or reserves. This policy meant that Aboriginal groups such as the Warlpiri, Pintupi, Luritja, Anmatyer, Pitjantjatjara, Kukatja, Arrernte and others were herded together to live away from their country, custom and sacred sites in the Northern Territory, creating major disruptions to and difficulties in Aboriginal lives. Since the 1970s, a government policy of self-determination has seen Aboriginal family groups return to traditional homelands, and the numbers of residents on some of the mission and reserve settlements have drastically reduced. For instance, Haast's Bluff, an Aboriginal reserve where over one thousand Aboriginal people resided in the 1950s, now has only about 180 Aboriginal residents (Ikuntji artists, 2010).

In desert Australia, there are three other smaller town settlements—Karratha, Port Hedland and Port Augusta—each with between 5000 and 17999 people; these two were settled predominantly by non-Aboriginal residents. The mining boom has meant that Aboriginal people living and working in Port Hedland, for instance, now find it difficult to obtain suitable housing, as house prices and rents have soared due to highly paid mining workers competing for scarce housing. Those people arriving in Port Hedland to work in the mines from around Australia who are unable to pay high rents may end up living in caravan parks, and even these have waiting lists (see Carney, 2008). The benefits derived from the mining boom are not necessarily shared locally with town residents or previous traditional owners of the land. Small local businesses also find it difficult to attract and retain workers, and a lack of affordable houses means local workers may end up moving elsewhere.

A further 29 settlements are located in desert Australia with between 1000 and 5000 residents and the Aboriginal population is also not predominant in these towns. There are rural towns of between 200 and 999 residents and small rural towns of 50 to 199 residents, which have a mixture of Aboriginal and non-Aboriginal residents—for instance, Birdsville, where Aboriginal people make up 33 per cent of the town's population out of a total of 112 residents (ABS, 2007c). Some local shires employ Aboriginal residents in a range of roles, including as road construction crew and community developers.

Governments have often flagged concerns about Aborigines camping within or just outside town boundaries, and official policy towards the 'town camps' in desert Australia has treated these settlements as 'illegal'. An historical understanding of these camps recognises that 'town camps' are the direct result of colonisation and the forced dispossession of Aboriginal people from their traditional lands, causing major disruptions of Aboriginal livelihood strategies. Governments have rarely or reluctantly provided minimal if any basic essential services like water, sanitation and public transport to these camps. Around Alice Springs in the 1970s, a group called Tangatijira—a local Aboriginal Arrernte word for 'working together'—was formed to assist Aboriginal people to gain some form of legal tenure of the land they were living on in order to obtain essential services and housing (Satour, 2009).

Generally, Aboriginal people live outside settled towns in desert Australia. The trend in desert Australia seems to be that the Aboriginal population is growing and the non-Aboriginal population tends to be declining (Davies & Holcombe, 2009). There are variations to this depending on the location of the place and the livelihood strategies—for instance, mining towns tend to reverse this trend. Another trend identified in desert Australia is the homelands movement, also called the outstation movement, where small communities with fewer than 50 people (usually comprising one or two Aboriginal families) are returning to traditional lands and caring for country in remote places away from other towns and settlements:

> In 2006, of the 93,000 Aboriginal and Torres Strait Islander peoples living in discrete Indigenous communities, nearly 33 per cent of people were in communities with less than 200 residents. The Northern Territory has the highest proportion of Indigenous people living in discrete communities, approximately 45 per cent, with 81 per cent of its Indigenous population living in remote or very remote areas. (AHRC, 2009)

165

There is significant diversity among various homeland settlements, with a range of livelihoods—some are focused on arts production, some on natural resource management, wildlife harvesting, teaching assistance, labouring on infrastructure initiatives like road building or maintenance, while others are more dependent on welfare income (Altman, 2009). The Northern Territory Intervention treated all homelands communities in the same manner, which failed to recognise the great variation between these homeland settlements. This indiscriminate approach meant resources were wasted through duplication or unnecessary provision of, for instance, health checks in one community, illustrated in Julie Nimmo and Tom Zubrycki's (2008) documentary, which focuses on the effects of the Intervention on four desert settlements in the Northern Territory.

THE HOMELANDS MOVEMENT IN DESERT AUSTRALIA

By the 1970s, it was clear that the assimilation policy was not working and it was officially abandoned by the Whitlam Labor government and replaced with the notion of Aboriginal community self-determination. This policy of self-determination facilitated the homelands movement, which has become so evident in desert Australia. The homelands movement was 'enabled through land rights and native title legislation and the infrastructure support that could be leveraged throughout the 1980s' (Young & Guenther, 2008: 178). The homelands movement has meant that Aboriginal people have been able to return to their traditional lands, and thus gain some reprieve from settlements that were created by missionaries or governments with little regard for Aboriginal culture, language, traditional lands, livelihoods and access to trade. The homelands movement is considered to facilitate 'a safer, healthier and culturally more satisfying lifestyle, free of the social stresses, alcohol abuse, petrol sniffing and domestic violence of some of the larger communities and towns' (McDermott et al., 1998; Young & Guenther, 2008: 178).

A quote from one of the homelands movement's leaders, Yananymul Mununggurr of Laynhapuy Homelands Association, in March 2009 highlights the significance of homelands:

Being in our Homelands, means that the land owns us, our identity comes from this land, our Homelands have stories behind them, which is done on bark paintings, sung in our song lines, danced in our dances; our language comes from this land, and the history of our land has been handed down generation after generation.

We are traditional people and we would like to keep it that way, we want our culture, language, identity to stay strong forever and at the same time we would like to adapt to that of mainstream Australia.

We are not moving from our Homelands, we are here to stay, we have rights to live and work in our Country; we are interconnected with each other and with our land. (AHRC, 2009)

Government policy and service-delivery methods can support and facilitate homelands movements, or they can have a significant negative impact. Social workers as policy-makers and analysts, researchers, community developers, service planners and providers play a role in supporting and facilitating Aboriginal self-determination and the provision of adequate resources to homeland communities. The provision of services in education, health, housing, support services and especially child protection are currently grossly underfunded, and require major commitment by governments and social workers to extend support to homelands communities to foster opportunities for homelands children to flourish (Northern Territory Government, 2010).

SERVICE DELIVERY AND GOVERNANCE

One of the mechanisms for service delivery and governance in remote homelands settlements over the last two decades has been the Homelands Resource Centres. These centres are Aboriginal community-controlled organisations that assist homelands communities with a range of technical and maintenance tasks. Some of these centres were also agencies for the Commonwealth-funded Community Development Employment Project (CDEP), which provided funding for community members to carry out tasks in the homelands (AHRC, 2009). Mostly these organisations focused on one single desert settlement, while regional organisations provided specific types of services, like health or legal assistance.

From the mid-1980s, the Northern Territory government encouraged multi-settlement incorporations, and by 2000 there were 68 local governing bodies spread across the Northern Territory. Aboriginal incorporations and councils have been very active in providing services to homelands through self-governance. The demands on these

Aboriginal local bodies in relation to delivering services for federal and territory governments are extensive and increasingly complex. According to Mark Moran and Ruth Elvin (2009), there have also been 'increasing demands on Aboriginal settlements for accountability and increases in complicated administrative instruments' for compliance with various levels of government and different government departments 'placing an enormous burden on the Aboriginal council to engage in a proliferation of administrative detail' (2009: 418–19). Moran and Elvin argue that the 'whole-of-government' coordinated trial in a remote settlement in the Northern Territory found that, as a result of the changes, 'rather than decreasing the quantity of administration, the number of funding programs increased from about 60 to 90' (Gray, 2006, cited in Moran & Elvin, 2009: 419). This greater complexity means that almost all of the senior positions in these local Aboriginal organisations are held by 'outsiders'—mostly non-Aboriginal people or Aboriginal people originally from elsewhere. Yet these roles require 'a high degree of local familiarity and trust' (Moran & Elvin, 2009: 419). Under the Northern Territory Intervention, community business managers were put in charge of Aboriginal communities to write funding submissions and garner resources for the community, without any previous connection with or knowledge of these communities (see Nimmo & Zubrycki, 2008).

VIABILITY OF THE HOMELANDS MOVEMENT

The homelands movement came under scrutiny by the former Howard Coalition government in 2005 when Amanda Vanstone, the then federal Indigenous Affairs Minister, indicated that she was not keen on homelands as they were 'cultural museums' that made white people feel good, but did not allow for Aboriginal people to have a viable future (Grill, 2006). The arguments against homelands settlements were around the difficulties these settlements posed for service delivery by the then-responsible Commonwealth government:

> A neoliberal commentary ensued, largely championed by the Bennelong Society, including the 'Leaving Remote Communities' conference in Sydney in September 2006, which appears to have had significant influence on policy. (Short, 2010: 60)

The survival of homelands as a sustainable livelihoods strategy for Aboriginal people is threatened by government policy through changes that transferred the responsibility for the delivery of essential and municipal services to homelands from the federal government to the Northern Territory government. With the introduction of the replacement of Aboriginal community councils with shire councils under the *Local Government Act* 2008, the Northern Territory government sought to amalgamate the incorporated community-based organisations based in desert regions of the Northern Territory. There was to be one municipality, Alice Springs, and three shires. This meant that small Aboriginal-incorporated community organisations were required to amalgamate across large geographic areas (Sanders & Holcombe, 2007), adding yet another layer of governance and complication to organising service delivery to homelands communities.

A further identified threat to homelands communities is the Council of Australian Governments (COAG) funding through partnership agreements between the federal government and the Northern Territory under the federal government's National Partnership Agreement on Remote Service Delivery, which has prioritised services in 26 selected sites in Australia, fifteen of which are in the Northern Territory (COAG, 2008, cited in AHRC, 2009):

> Much of the funding commitment made through such COAG agreements is for prioritised, larger, Indigenous communities, with comparatively lower levels of resources and service provision being made available in other, smaller, communities, many of which are homeland communities. (AHRC, 2009)

Damien Short (2010) considers that 'with this new "Working Future" initiative, the Northern Territory government is now seeking to urbanize those remaining indigenous peoples living in remote communities by moving financial support away from outstations to twenty larger Aboriginal communities' "Territory Growth Towns"' (2010: 60). A neo-liberal paradigm informs the 'Working Future' policy statement in that these towns are to focus 'sustainable economic development' in desert Australia. According to Jon Altman (2009: n.p.), there is an alternative that is worthy of 'serious policy consideration'. He suggests that the Northern Territory government support 'the aspirations and determination of outstation people to live on their land pursuing a way of life that incorporates two ways: the customary and the market, Aboriginal and European'. There is:

a growing body of research [that] has indicated that life at out-stations is better—in health outcomes, livelihood options, and social cohesion, even housing conditions—than at larger townships, despite neglect . . . Many Aboriginal people remain determined to live on their ancestral lands, pursuing a way of life that is informed by fundamentally different value systems. (Altman, 2009: n.p.)

Social workers from an anti-racist and anti-oppressive theoreti-cal perspective are positioned to take Aboriginal people's desires to remain on country seriously, and work on research and policy advo-cacy that promotes adequate resourcing to redress the structural disadvantages experienced by Aboriginal people on homelands, in town camps and in small rural towns in desert Australia. Neo-liberal and conservative claims that land does not mean anything if Aborigi-nal people cannot thrive and attain 'real' jobs and gain proper quali-fications are only relevant if adequate resources and service delivery are developed so that Aboriginal people have the same rights and opportunities to thrive and flourish as other Australians without having to leave their homelands.

There are really strong arguments for anti-racist social workers to understand the links between Aboriginal people's well-being and their attachment to land in desert Australia (Short, 2010). The effect of colonisation in Australia has forced Aboriginal people to be displaced from their relationship with the land, and the inter-connection of loss of land, livelihood and cultural practices has led to 'community-wide trauma and dysfunction' (Short, 2010: 52). Social workers are aware of the broader context of Aboriginal colo-nisation, particularly past government policies of so-called 'protec-tion' and assimilation recorded in the *Bringing Them Home* report (HREOC, 1997). The inquiry into the effects of the government policy of removing Aboriginal children from their families—often forcibly—showed that these policies and actions had caused great harm to Aboriginal people; indeed, the policy was termed genocide by Sir Ronald Wilson, one of the authors of the report. There is a strong argument from an anti-oppressive and anti-racist social work perspective for recognising and restoring Aboriginal land rights and self-determination as a way of working towards decolonising rela-tions in Australia.

Aboriginal children taken from their families and placed in insti-tutions or with white families were removed from their culture, language, traditional knowledge, liberty, dignity and identity. There was further trauma as some of these stolen Aboriginal children suffered physical and sexual abuse at the hands of their out-of-home carers while official bodies failed to protect them (HREOC, 1997). Judy Atkinson's (2002) work on trauma trails and the cross-generational impact of colonisation and dispossession is an excellent resource to assist social workers' understanding of and response to the effects of these multiple losses.

In 2008, Prime Minister Kevin Rudd 'apologised for the hurt, pain, suffering, indignity, degradation and humiliation caused by successive parliaments' (T. Smith, 2008: n.p.). The Australian Association of Social Workers 'endorsed a statement of apology on behalf of the Australian Social Welfare Sector' in 1997, and made a formal apology to the stolen generation (Calma, 2008: n.p.). A joint media release from the National Coalition of Aboriginal and Torres Strait Islander Social Workers Association (NCATSISWA) and the Australian Association of Social Workers (AASW) and other social work peak bodies, put out in response to the Northern Territory Intervention, states:

> The experience of the Stolen Generations has taught us that well-intentioned Interventions with children and families can have long term consequences. Social workers have acknowledged with regret the part we have played in that policy and we are determined that it should not happen again. Long term solutions can only be found by working closely and respectfully with Indigenous communities. (Calma, 2008: n.p.)

Short (2010) argues that the recent Northern Territory Intervention is a continuation of the earlier policies of colonialism and genocide, and regards this legislation as continuing the suffering, indignity, degradation and humiliation of Aboriginal people.

THE NORTHERN TERRITORY INTERVENTION

The *Little Children Are Sacred* report (Wild & Anderson, 2007) stated that the situation in some Northern Territory Aboriginal communities was due to the 'breakdown of indigenous culture and society, as a consequence of colonial dispossession and the combined effects of poor health, alcohol and drug abuse, unemployment and poor education and housing' (Short, 2010: 56). The report made recommendations for a whole range of changes in relation to unemployment, education, health and alcohol consumption, and was very clear on the point that Aboriginal communities were to be empowered 'to take more control and to make their own decisions about their future' (Short, 2010: 56). Yet this most important aspect of the report's recommendations was overridden in the rush to protect children—a laudable goal, but more than three years after the introduction of the Intervention, the expected increase in the reporting of child sexual abuse has not occurred (see Nimmo & Zubrycki, 2008).

Despite the 'emergency' response to child sexual abuse in remote Australian communities, child sexual abuse is not often reported for Aboriginal children in the Northern Territory (Northern Territory Government, 2010). Child neglect is the more commonly substantiated claim, which is consistent with the disadvantaged socio-economic conditions evident in many Aboriginal communities, including over-crowded housing, low levels of employment opportunities and a lack of social services (Northern Territory Government, 2010).

The Northern Territory Intervention has had a major impact on Aboriginal communities' livelihoods through the raft of changes introduced, including the abolition of the CDEP scheme, the suspension of the *Race Discrimination Act* 1975, the quarantining of 50 per cent of Centrelink income and the compulsory takeover of Aboriginal towns—which also means that community leaders no longer have a say over local projects. The CDEP scheme provided a revenue stream for more than 200 Aboriginal organisations in remote desert settlements, and before the intervention about 7500 Aboriginal people were employed by the scheme. There were more than 500 CDEP participants working in Northern Territory schools, according to the Australian Education Union (AEU), as teacher assistants, home liaison officers, bilingual literacy workers (keeping in mind that English is a second if not third language for many desert Aboriginal people), bus drivers and cultural teachers. These CDEP positions were not turned into 'real' jobs. Only sixteen new full-time employment positions were created, and these were classified at the lowest level in the Northern Territory public sector: 'All of the positions were cut in half and at 0.5 the wage is less than $16 000 per annum. Many ex-CDEP workers have not accepted this "demotion" and are now unemployed' (Gibson, 2010: 6). The impact of this policy on Aboriginal young people has been particularly harsh for those living on homelands, as they have to be in employment or enrolled in school, VET or with a Registered Training Organisation (RTO) to be eligible for any benefits. The Australian Education Union estimates that 3000 young Aborigines are likely to be affected, without any hope of gaining employment (Gibson, 2010: 8).

To introduce Income Management, which quarantines 50 per cent of all the Centrelink entitlements received by Aboriginal people, required the suspension of the *Racial Discrimination Act 1975*. It was not possible to quarantine CDEP wages, because these were paid through the CDEP providers, the homelands resource centres or councils. Aboriginal people had to be moved off CDEP to have their incomes managed by Centrelink. These policies leave few choices to Aboriginal people, who have lost both employment and income. The effect of the Northern Territory Intervention has been to push people to leave their homeland communities for urban centres, and this is creating major issues in

> already overcrowded town camps and the under-resourced Aboriginal organisations. Not surprisingly these changes to Aboriginal peoples' livelihoods [are] creating stress and Family, Housing, Community Services and Indigenous Affairs (FAHCSIA, 2009) indicated that incidents of domestic violence are up 61%, substance abuse up 77% and 13% more infants are being hospitalised since the start of the Northern Territory Emergency Intervention. (Gibson, 2010: 11)

CASE STUDY

Imagine you are a social worker in Alice Springs and a young Aboriginal person arrives from a homelands setting to find employment and housing in town.

Reflective questions

- What are the issues confronting this young person?
- What resources would you be able to offer?
- With whom would you want to connect this young person?
- On what policy advocacy would you work?
- Which organisations might you join to attempt to effect change?
- What community development projects would you advocate for with the local shire, the Northern Territory government and non-government organisations, and how would you get involved with Aboriginal organisations to improve service delivery?

A social worker informed by an anti-oppressive theoretical perspective focuses their practice on three levels: the individual person; their community and local services; and the policy advocacy level. Social workers need to work interprofessionally with others in the community and government to effect changes in policy, to improve service provision and to design community development projects with the people affected by these policies. Social workers in remote Aboriginal settlements have been positioned as part of the problem through previous and current government policies and practices. An adequate response to this positioning means facing this uncomfortable place by not withdrawing out of fear of making things worse. This means not buying into the ongoing institutional racism that accepts lower conditions of living for Aboriginal people in homelands, town camps or some remote desert towns.

SUMMARY

The emphasis in this book on livelihood strategies in rural and remote areas of Australia relates to the importance of income security, stable and affordable housing, accessible health care, good-quality and relevant schooling and a diversity of food sources as a 'fundamental basis for a preventive approach to child protection' in the homelands (Northern Territory Government, 2010). One of the key challenges for social workers is working out how to engage in developing 'community-driven service design' within the context of the Northern Territory government where there is an absence of capacity to provide effective family and support services (2010: 33). The *Bringing Them Home* report (HREOC, 1997) presents many tragic testimonials of the failure of care provided by the state and various institutions. This means that social workers working in rural and remote desert Australia are called on to engage with the challenge of designing, developing and providing support services in collaboration with Aboriginal communities and families. The stakes are very high, and many of the policies that have recently been introduced by the Northern Territory and federal governments make it far more difficult for Aboriginal families to stay on country and use the homelands lifestyle to promote a sense of well-being. The challenge for social workers is to engage with the impact of these wider policies on livelihood strategies, and to work with communities on designing service delivery while being sensitive to the significant diversity among homelands communities.

RECOMMENDED READING

Langton, M. & Perkins, R. (eds) (2008) *First Australians: An illustrated history*. Melbourne University Press, Melbourne.

Resources related to homelands and Aboriginal rights can be found at: <www.ourgeneration.org.au/resources/>.

12

ENGAGING WITH SEA-CHANGE AND TREE-CHANGE FAMILIES OVER TIME

Sarah Wendt

CHAPTER OBJECTIVES

- To explore the experiences of different age groups within families living in a rural setting, particularly focusing on farming families.
- To learn how systems and feminist theory can help social workers understand some of the impacts of environmental changes on individual family members.
- To consider how policy and service frameworks impact on families living in rural settings.
- To learn how systems and feminist theory inform solution-focused methods of practice when working directly with families living in rural settings.

INTRODUCTION

It is not possible to come up with a standard definition of family due to the many and varied households that exist today (parents with children, couples with no children, single-parent families, extended family, grandparents, gay and lesbian couples, adopted or fostered children, and so on). Generally, a family can be considered any group of individuals who live together and who are expected to perform specific functions, especially in relation to children (Ambrosino et al., 2008). This chapter provides an overview of living in a rural community from the perspectives of different members who make up a family.

Change impacting on rural communities in Australia comes from movements such as the sea-changers/tree-changers. Sea-changers and tree-changers are families that move to coastal or forested places, which often offer beautiful natural surroundings. These locations are away from major cities, and this can impact on the needs of different family members over time. This chapter argues that systems theory, coupled with feminist theory, can provide useful insights into understanding the impact of such changes on families, particularly farming families. This chapter also outlines a solution-focused framework as a method for providing direction for social workers' interventions when working with the individual members who make up families.

FAMILIES OVER TIME

When asked to describe a family living in a rural place, most people would imagine mum, dad and a number of children living on a farming property. In fact, rural regions and populations—as well as industries—are diverse, and so are the families that make up rural communities. Ruth Panelli (2006) points out that the family has long been a unit of inquiry and analysis in rural studies, especially through the investigations of farming or community life, and so for the purposes of this chapter, farming families are a good place to begin. Farming families have been selected because, as Alston (2009a) states, many people are linked to farms and agricultural development in Australia. Australian agriculture is predominantly based on a family farming model, with over 90 per cent of farms run by families, rising to 99 per cent in broad acres and dairy farming (Alston, 2009a: 134). Families make up a significant part of rural economies, employment bases, and population in rural communities. Farms are diverse and include small horticultural ventures, boutique wineries, niche market foods, dairy, broad acre cropping, livestock, and large cattle stations (Alston, 2009a).

Children, youth, men and women, and older people all experience living in rural communities differently. Research has looked at how rurality impacts on people's lives across the lifespan. This is a helpful starting point to generally outline what it is like to grow up and live in a rural community.

For children, rural communities are often represented as places of fun, adventure and freedom because of the opportunity to explore physical environments and engage in activities such as learning how to fish or catch yabbies, climbing haystacks, and watching the births of animals. Furthermore, rural communities are cited as 'safe places' to bring up children, and this is often a reason given by families who migrate to rural areas. People often say things like: 'You don't have to lock your door' or 'Children can go down the street on their own', which indicates that rural places are often constructed as environments that offer safety from crime and other hazards such as traffic that come from urban spaces (Woods, 2005). However, at the same time children experience contradictions to these images of freedom, exploration and safety because of isolation, distance and transportation restrictions. Catching up with friends after school or on weekends may be difficult, as this often requires transportation to different towns, villages or farms. Children may also experience restrictions on activities such as sport and leisure due to limited public transport, high fuel costs and dependency on mum or dad for transport (Woods, 2005).

For young people, research has generally looked at how rurality impacts on their leisure and educational opportunities. Youth in rural communities often express a sense of amenity deprivation when they compare their lives with those of urban youth. It is not uncommon to hear them say 'There is nothing for young people to do' as an expression of frustration at the limited shops, leisure outlets and entertainment facilities. Despite this, the diversity and number of leisure activities focusing on physical sports, such as football and cricket, are indicative of many rural communities (Fabiansson, 2006). However, it is also important to note that rural communities are more likely to support and cater for young males than for young females when it comes to sport, and young people not interested in physical sports often face a void in suitable leisure and recreational activities (Fabiansson, 2006).

The shortage of recreational facilities and the associated frustration and sense of boredom are often identified as contributing factors to problems such as under-age drinking, drug abuse and vandalism in rural areas (Woods, 2005). Similarly, tensions can grow in rural communities as young people gather in public spaces such as parks, shopping centres and school grounds, which can be perceived as threatening by other residents (Woods, 2005).

Despite such criticisms or tensions experienced by young people, many want to remain in their home area; however, job and education opportunities are often limited. For example, pursuing higher education commonly means leaving your rural community and attending an institution in the city. Families face many obstacles when they decide to support a young person to pursue education or employment opportunities away from home. Finance is a factor where families are faced with the high costs of study and relocating, as well as the material costs associated with living away from home. Other obstacles include the anxiety about safety and loneliness felt by the young person who decides to move away from home. It is not uncommon for young people to feel 'homesick' when they leave their communities and families for education purposes, due to the close-knit nature of many communities and the tight bonds between family members (Alloway & Dalley-Trim, 2009).

Young people who don't leave their communities for education or employment opportunities are often faced with restricted local labour market opportunities, which can be poorly paid, provide insecure positions and offer few opportunities for career advancement. Such things can make it difficult for young people to obtain affordable housing of their own (Woods, 2005).

Older people living in rural communities have different experiences. Active engagement in the agricultural workforce often gives rural people not only income but also social standing where they live. However, retirement from the workforce raises a number of issues. For example, the change in economic capacity and transfer to 'beneficiary' status can separate older people (particularly farming men) from mainstream life in rural places (Chalmers & Joseph, 2006). Competently managing and protecting assets to provide a retirement income and choices in housing, health and community care as people age can bring stress and worry to older people, especially when they are trying to please all family members (Tilse et al., 2006).

Despite this departure from the workforce, older people often become consumers too, with rural lifestyles drawing locals and newcomers to buy property or enter retirement villages and consume local amenities and services (Chalmers & Joseph, 2006). However, older people can also be faced with broader changes in provision systems. For example, when rural communities experience closure of banks, shops and services, this can create flow-on problems with mobility and transportation issues, and increase the costs of living. Older people can also be faced with the adoption of new technologies, such as telecommunications, the internet and digital technology. These advances impact on vital banking and postal services (on which older people are heavily reliant), and consequently older people can feel excluded by and from the pervasive introduction of new technology into rural places (Woods, 2005; Chalmers & Joseph, 2006). Ageing also increases physical and mental limitations and/ or disability (Chalmers & Joseph, 2006). Depending on the rural community in which they live, older people can be faced with limited access to health services and/or mobility restrictions as a result of the physical environment, making the loss of independence more problematic. Yet, by living rurally, older people can at times have access to local specialised ageing services that are supported by informal community networks built on strong social capital (Woods, 2005).

When looking at families in rural communities, gender cannot be ignored. Alston (2005a) argues that the division of labour, uneven power relations and the profile of rural landholders and business owners, as well as holders of public office, voluntary workers and child carers, all show that gender is a critical determinant of the lived experience of rural communities. She maintains that hegemonic masculinity is clearly evident in rural Australian communities when we look at the institutional structures, such as law and religion, and the processes and practices, such as patrilineal inheritance, through which gender relations are constructed and reconstructed in everyday life. As a consequence, masculinist understandings of rural community life are privileged, with many sites of masculine power and privilege displayed in public spaces in rural communities, such as farm organisations, local government, pubs, livestock yards and playing fields for male-dominated sports. Consequently, female-dominated public spaces are often limited; they include health centres, schools, church halls and gathering spaces to do craft and for fundraising. Generally, women are more socially inclusive and community focused, and so tend to maintain a community's social capital structures to a higher extent than males (Fabiansson, 2006).

CHANGES IMPACTING ON FAMILIES

Overall, rural population characteristics mirror national trends, such as an ageing population, smaller families, increasing family diversity and higher divorce rates. However, distinct trends can also be identified in rural settings, and changes in population trends and global pressures have unique impacts on farming families. For example, in recent years we have seen the long-running drought and declining water availability across Australia. These issues have significantly impacted rural communities, bringing social effects such as health and welfare implications, levels of poverty and declining access to education and employment opportunities (Alston, 2009a). Pugh and Cheers (2010: 10) point out that the reduction in traditional forms of employment, together with changing aspirations, has led to young people and younger families leaving rural areas, resulting in a shift towards an older population in rural communities because people of working age and school-leavers often seek employment and education elsewhere.

To understand these changes in more detail, we can look at a recent trend being acknowledged in Australia: the emergence of the 'sea-changers' and 'tree-changers'.

SEA-CHANGERS/TREE-CHANGERS

Economic globalisation, combined with the pressures described above, has created enormous wealth in the cities, and this is now being expressed directly and indirectly in demand for the material and amenity resources of rural regions, such as new wine-production areas and revitalised domestic tourism economies (Alston, 2009a; Burnley & Murphy, 2004). The global pressures have influenced a phenomenon known as the 'sea-change' or 'tree-change'. These terms generally refer to the movement of Australians from metropolitan cities to non-metropolitan parts of the country. The predominant reason for this move has been the search for a low-key lifestyle away from the high costs and high pressures faced in big cities (Burnley & Murphy, 2004).

When we think about sea-changers or tree-changers, our imaginations often move towards affluence—for example, high-income earners who have investment incomes or high-paying occupations that do not require them to be at city workplaces on a regular basis, or who can obtain elevated incomes in non-metropolitan areas (Burnley & Murphy, 2004). We also think of retirees who are searching for the benefits of trading down from high-priced city houses to cheaper or higher quality housing, as well as the attractions of low-key lifestyles in a high-amenity environment. Retirees often go back to where they were born or to places about which they have extensive knowledge due to previous holidays and even ownership of second homes. Other more affluent sea-changers and tree-changers are those who move from the city to make a good living servicing retirees and tourists, or who continue to travel and work in city locations but at the same time experience cheaper housing (Burnley & Murphy, 2004).

Ian Burnley and Peter Murphy (2004) also point out that it is important not to forget that lower-income people also move to rural places in Australia in search of affordable housing—especially those relying on income-support payments. Broadly speaking, then, sea-changers or tree-changers are those who more or less make a free choice to leave cities compared with those who to some extent are pushed out of the city because of the high costs of living (Burnley & Murphy, 2004), but they are also people with incomes that are too low to enable them to live in appropriate and affordable housing. These people often rely on some form of income-support payment (Burnley & Murphy, 2004).

This shift has been seen in many other Western industrialised nations, and is also known as a 'population turnaround' (Burnley & Murphy, 2004; Kelly & Hosking, 2008). This shift creates the basis for demographic, economic and social changes in non-metropolitan areas, and impacts on families because it raises challenges for land use, infrastructure, local cultures of places and a sense of community (Burnley & Murphy, 2004).

USING SYSTEMS AND FEMINIST THEORY TO UNDERSTAND HOW CHANGE IMPACTS ON FAMILIES

All families have strengths and different ways of coping with change. In the 1970s, Urie Bronfenbrenner emphasised the importance of understanding the developing person in the context of the family, social network, community and wider society. He highlighted the importance of recognising different contexts in which people are embedded (Scott et al., 2010). For example, human development can be conceptualised within a concentric arrangement of the following systems, and analysing each system level provides different insights (Munford et al., 2005; Ambrosino et al., 2008; Scott et al., 2010).

Microsystem

The microsystem is the smallest and most direct system that a person experiences; it includes all persons and groups that incorporate a person's day-to-day environment, such as family, workplace, friends and church. At this level of analysis, the social worker aims to gain an idea of the social relationships in the person's life. Social capital maintains ties between individuals, and shows relationships between relatives and close friends, and within social groups, which can reveal various other attributes, such as trust, reciprocity and shared values and norms, altruism, shared beliefs, tolerance, a sense of belonging to a community, self-reliance and self-help (Dibden & Cocklin, 2005).

Mesosystem

The mesosystem shows the interrelationships between two or more microsystems, as well as the extent to which experiences are reinforcing or conflictual. The stronger and more diverse the links are between microsystems, the more positive influence the mesosystem has upon the developing person. For example, it can show the social worker how home life impacts on the workplace, or how church impacts on family life. Exploring relationships between microsystems can potentially show where 'tensions' and 'stresses', or 'fit' and 'equilibrium', are experienced by someone in their environment (Ambrosino et al., 2008).

Exosystem

The exosystem includes one or more settings that do not involve the developing person as a direct participant, but nonetheless may have an influence on them. For example, policies on parental leave in a parent's workplace can influence the time a child spends with their working parent. Or the attitudes and beliefs emanating from the local football club can influence whether a young person plays sport. The exosystem can be thought of as the community level, and focuses on factors that may not relate directly to the person but affects the way in which they function. For example, local community values and attitudes can impact on individuals. While closely knit communities tend to have strong informal networks based on friendships and family ties, and are positive features of this social organisation, these attributes may also obstruct anonymity and confidentiality, thereby making it more difficult for people to seek assistance with a range of social issues (violence and abuse, mental health, financial assistance, and so on) (Wendt, 2009).

The exosystem provides a social worker with a strong place to start their analysis because it reveals particular details about a rural community, such as the geographic area (names of roads, terrain, distance), the demographics of the place (age, ethnicity, income of residents), local culture (politics, religions, informal networks, civic groups) and community leaders and information resources (including religious organisations, community, civic and service groups, and informal community nurturers and supporters). The exosystem allows social workers to gain a strong understanding of the community and its qualities and stories, and provides insight into how it may be possible to work together in positive ways. Gaining an appreciation of the community ultimately builds a better position to construct helping activities and relationships tailored to individual people and families (the microsystems) that make up rural communities (Wendt, 2009).

Macrosystem

The macrosystem encapsulates the wider social policy, socio-cultural settings and institutional life of the society. It includes the ideological, customary and legal norms, social policy, social ideology and values, legislation and government, as well as the natural environment. It influences all the other levels of the environment and can be considered the over-arching cultural blueprint of a society. The macrosystem allows the social worker to explore the broad values of a society, to see which groups are more oppressed by other groups, and to ask how this would personally impact on a person. Similarly, the social worker can explore what state or federal policies or institutional structures are directly influencing individuals (Dibden & Cocklin, 2005; Ambrosino et al., 2008), or ask how a drought or water restrictions—the natural environment—may be impacting on families.

Systems theory can be used to investigate how a range of environmental changes can affect rural families because it provides a framework for understanding complex interactions between groups of people. It particularly draws attention to the multiple systems within which people function, and enables the social worker to contextually situate people within their specific environment (Ambrosino et al., 2008). It identifies a wide range of factors that impact on social welfare problems, and shifts attention solely from the characteristics of individuals or the environment to the transactions *between* systems—that is, the focus becomes the person in environment. Social workers can target intervention at a variety of levels to address social problems and individual needs (Ambrosino et al., 2008).

Although systems theory provides a detailed starting point for social workers to grasp contexts within which people live and to customise interventions for individuals who make up families, the theory falls short in its acknowledgement of notions of power, oppression and marginalisation. With such a heavy focus on people and their environment, a critique of power is often overlooked. To supplement systems theory, critical theories can help to further analyse rural families and examine how change impacts on different members. Critical theories focus on structural rather than personal explanations of social problems, together with a concern for inequality and oppression (Payne, 2005). Oppression in its various forms becomes a central organising theme used to analyse domination of some groups in society by other groups, including how such domination is sustained through structural processes (McDonald, 2006). As a social worker, this prompts one to recognise social processes associated with class, race, age and gender, as well as other social categories.

In particular, feminist theory provides an effective supplement to systems theory because it picks up a focus on gender differences. Gender needs to feature in discussions about families, in which power imbalances can be manifested at a range of levels, from the interpersonal through to the institutional and societal (Fawcett & Waugh, 2008). For example, men are more likely to work full time, hold public positions of power and occupy public spaces in rural communities, whereas women are more likely to have significant responsibility for household and care work, to work part time, and to undertake community and volunteer work (Alston, 2005a). Feminist theory allows for an examination of the gendered experiences of living in a rural community, and how power operates within gender relations.

Rural community studies have revealed that masculine hegemony is highly resistant to change, though it is important to also recognise that some resistance by women is also evident (Alston, 2005a; Wendt, 2009). Lia Bryant and Barbara Pini (2011) encourage the examination of power in rural spaces, and the diversity and multiplicity of oppressions, resistance and agency. They argue that gender and rurality cannot be examined in isolation from other social locations, and so interrogate categories such as 'rural woman' and 'rural man' to explore the ways in which gender coexists and melds with indigeneity, ethnicity, class, sexuality, disability and age. Bryant and Pini reject totalising claims about male dominance and female subordination, instead arguing that at particular times and in specific spaces, inequalities are produced and contested between women and men, and further, between groups of women and groups of men.

POLICY AND SERVICE FRAMEWORKS IMPACTING ON FAMILIES OVER TIME

The Australian federal and state governments aim to provide policies and services that specifically assist families living in rural communities. A good preparation task before working in a rural community as a social worker is to explore the current policies/services that impact on families. It is also important to gain an understanding of the global and national economic and social changes specifically impacting on families in rural communities. This chapter goes some way towards providing a starting point for this.

However, it is also important for social workers working in rural contexts to bring their critical theory lens with them when examining policy because not all policies formed (even with the best intentions) by government necessarily translate easily into rural practice contexts. Brian Cheers and Judy Taylor (2005) argue that mainstream welfare policies, structures and methods have been extended to rural areas over the last few decades in an attempt to respond to rural needs, but many of their inadequacies have been exposed. Urban-based central Commonwealth and state governments, rather than local government and community-based organisations, have separated social policy formulation and service provision from the communities in which people live. Consequently, central government domination, concerns about consistency of service standards and the urban foundations of Australian welfare have contributed to the adoption of uniform service approaches that tend to be unresponsive or confusing for different geographical, social and cultural contexts of rural communities in Australia (Cheers & Taylor, 2005).

As an example of Cheers and Taylor's (2005) argument, Alston (2009a) points out that farming families in particular traditionally have been excluded from poverty-alleviation payments as a result of their assets base, so addressing farming poverty is complex. The main measure designed to give farm household support is available through Exceptional Circumstances Relief Payments and the Exceptional Circumstances Interest Rate Subsidy to assist with the costs of drought livestock feeding and transport costs. However, a family cannot seek funding under these schemes unless their area has been declared by the government to be in exceptional circumstances.

Once the declaration is made, it can take months to apply for the support and for it to be assessed and granted (Alston, 2009a). Similarly, assets-based criteria have often meant that rural young people applying for Youth Allowance to study away from home are excluded from receiving such financial support. It is worth noting that in April 2010, the Rudd Labor government implemented reforms to student income support, especially for rural and remote students, and consequently parental income test cut-out points are now higher. Since January 2011, young people from rural areas who are required to relocate for study because of the geographic location of their family home are eligible to apply for assistance under a range of criteria.

Alston (2009a) argues that policy for farm families has been ad hoc and ill-considered, and has resulted in growing alienation and poverty among them. The complex process of policy, assessment times, complexity of asset valuation and determination, and a sense that families should be able to manage on their own often result in farming families receiving little support.

METHODS OF PRACTICE FOR WORKING WITH FAMILIES OVER TIME

Systems theory provides an overall way of describing things at any level, but it does not tell us what to do or where, or how to affect systems (Payne, 2005: 158). One method of practice for intervention with families that complements systems and feminist theory is solution-focused practice. This is a short-term approach to intervention in which the social worker and the client attend to solutions to problems more than they do to the problems themselves. Like systems theory, it assumes that human behaviour is predominantly learned in one's family of origin and the environment, and that activity in any area of a system affects all other areas (Walsh, 2010: 231). Walsh points out that because systems and solution-focused practice share these assumptions, a client's change efforts do not need to be related directly to a presenting problem because any change will affect the entire system and new actions will influence its elements in ways that cannot be predicted or contained. The social worker may thus consider many creative strategies for change when working with a client system (Walsh, 2010: 234).

There are specific intervention guidelines in solution-focused practice that complement feminist ways of working which a social worker can also use to work with different family members living in rural settings (Walsh, 2010):

- Be a collaborator—that is, collaborate with the client in defining their goals, and selecting goals and strategies that are achievable.
- Help people identify and amplify their strengths and resources to the goal of finding solutions to presenting problems.
- Discover exceptions to the client's problems and build solutions from such knowledge.
- Provide hope and support, communicate possibility of change, motivate and look to the future.

Such guidelines are similar to the values and principles of feminist practice, including working with social relationships in a holistic manner, linking women, men and children with their communities, focusing on capacities, strengths and skills, and focusing on connectedness and collaboration with others when finding solutions to problems (Payne, 2005).

CASE STUDY

The Ryan family lives in a rural community with a population of approximately 20 000, located an hour and a half from the nearest capital city. John works as a cereal crop farmer on his property. He is a fifth-generation farmer on the inherited property. The family earns a moderate income of $60 000 annually from the farm. Janet, John's wife, works on the farm with John and also works part-time as a cleaner for the local pub.

Janet and John attend church regularly, and Janet volunteers at the football canteen stall on most Saturdays. Over the last five years, the population of the region has increased significantly. Janet and John often talk to their neighbours and friends about the potential housing supply and cost for their children and ageing parents, as well as the destruction of the natural environment. The local families frequently talk about the newcomers being 'strangers', and believe they are not making an effort to engage with community activities because many are travelling to the city for work and leisure.

John and Janet have a seventeen-year-old-daughter, Alison, who is finishing high school and plans to study property law. Alison is feeling nervous and frightened about leaving home to study. They also have two sons, Thomas, aged fifteen, and Daniel, aged twelve. Thomas enjoys playing football and hopes to work on the farm, whereas Daniel enjoys computers and playing video games with his friends. They are extremely pleased that Thomas plans to work on the farm but are concerned that if Daniel expresses such an interest, they will not be able to financially support the employment of both sons. Daniel and Thomas have different interests, yet they are competitive, and John and Janet don't want to be seen as favouring one over the other. John and Janet are greatly concerned that they will not be able to financially support each of their children in the years to come while they are pursuing study and employment opportunities. Finally, John's mother, Joyce, is 75 years old and lives in a house approximately fifteen kilometres from the farm. She is a widow and is experiencing the onset of dementia. John and Janet know little about this health issue and worry about her safety.

Reflective questions

- Social workers are encouraged to examine power as part of their practice. In what ways would recognising social processes associated with class, race, age and gender, along with other social categories, aid a social worker working with the Ryan family?
- How can a social worker use micro, meso, exo and macro levels of systems theory to formulate different responses to the Ryan family's concerns? How might feminist theory further enhance the social worker's understanding of and response to the Ryan family?

SUMMARY

Rural families are extremely important to Australia's economy and broader identity. Change is experienced differently by children, young people, men and women, and older people living in rural communities, so it is important to continue to develop, refine and maintain services, policies and infrastructure to support families living in rural contexts. Systems theory and feminist theory both provide social workers with a map to help them understand rural contexts and some direction to assist them to provide support and advocacy to address the well-being of different family members. Solution-focused practice gives social workers specific guidelines so they can focus their interventions with individual family members.

RECOMMENDED READING

Alston, M. (2010) *Innovative Human Services Practice: Australia's changing landscape*. Palgrave Macmillan, Melbourne.

Bryant, L. & Pini, B. (2011) *Gender and Rurality*. Routledge, New York.

Cheers, B., Darracott, R. & Lonne, B. (2007) *Social Care Practice in Rural Communities*. Federation Press, Sydney.

Cocklin, C. & Dibden, J. (eds) (2005) *Sustainability and Change in Rural Australia*. UNSW Press, Sydney.

Pugh, R. & Cheers, B. (2010) *Rural Social Work: An international perspective*. Policy Press, Bristol.

Wendt, S. (2009), *Domestic Violence in Rural Australia*. Federation Press, Sydney.

Woods, M. (2005) *Rural Geography*. Sage, London.

13

FACILITATING INTERGENERATIONAL DIALOGUE: AGEING IN RURAL PLACES

Jeni Warburton and Suzanne Hodgkin

CHAPTER OBJECTIVES

- To provide an understanding of the broad issues facing Australia's ageing population and the current policy response to this.
- To provide a contextualised discussion of the current challenges facing older people living in rural and remote areas.
- To introduce concepts and approaches for social work practice with older rural people.

INTRODUCTION

Despite the many challenges facing older people living in regional and remote areas, this area of social work practice is seldom addressed in the practice literature. Recent and ongoing problems associated with globalisation, climate change and drought, and changes in family structure have impacted on the experience of growing older in the bush. This chapter examines these changes and identifies issues that need to inform rural social work practice.

AGEING CONTEXT AND POLICY

Australia, like most countries, has an ageing population. At the 2006 national Census, of just over 20 million people in Australia, 3.7 per cent of the population were aged 80 and over (termed the Oldest Generation); 14.5 per cent were aged 60–79 (the Lucky Generation); and 27.5 per cent were aged 40–59 (the Baby Boomer Generation) (ABS, 2006). It is the large size of the Baby Boomer Generation, now approaching retirement, that has skewed the population pyramid and led to serious concerns about the 'greying' of the population.

The age structure of the population has changed dramatically and steadily over the last century, with the proportion of those who are children declining from 35 to 20 per cent over the century, while the proportion of those aged 65 years and over has increased from 4 to 13 per cent. These changes reflect improvements in life expectancy due to better health care, nutrition and sanitation, as well as an accompanying decline in fertility rates (ABS, 2006).

These population changes have resulted in a number of challenges for the Australian government, particularly associated with the financing of such dramatic population change. As the population ages, concerns are growing about the shrinking size of the working population and their tax income in relation to the larger pool of those outside paid work. Termed the dependency ratio, this assumes that those outside paid work are dependent on those in paid work, and that there will be insufficient income to support them. This scenario has led to ageing being viewed as a potential social and economic crisis for future generations.

This is a simplistic assumption, however, and can be disputed on a number of levels. The notion of dependency in many cases is disputable, as many older people contribute to society, both within and outside paid work. Many give their time as volunteers, carers or to their communities, and without them many services simply would not exist (Warburton & McLaughlin, 2005).

In response to concerns about the ageing population, the Australian government is implementing new policies aimed at extending the working lives of people and keeping them in paid work for longer. These policies include changes to superannuation laws to encourage people to defer retirement, as well as reducing the numbers of those reliant on government pensions. For example, in the 2009 federal Budget, it was signalled that the pension age would be raised to 67 years. However, these policies appear to be unsuccessful to date, with little evidence of large numbers of people putting off retirement. Concerns about the costs of ageing are still at the forefront of the policy context.

The costs of an ageing population have been the focus of a series of key policy documents issued by the Australian Treasury, the

Intergenerational Reports, 2002–03, 2007 and 2009. Generally, these reports highlight concerns about the increased health costs associated with an ageing population. To mitigate these costs, the Australian government has moved towards promoting the notion of building healthy and active ageing. The result has been an emphasis on health promotion and community programs encouraging the involvement of older people in physical activity, learning new skills, and so on. The burgeoning of interest in men's sheds is a prime example of healthy and active ageing.

Australia is not alone in its emphasis on healthy and active ageing. Policy trends across the world are similarly focusing on how the health of the older population can be maintained. Certainly ageing is emerging as a serious concern for a number of countries with large populations, such as China. The World Health Organization issued a global active ageing policy in 2002, emphasising the three tiers of health, participation and security. As a result, the policy focus in a number of countries, including Australia, is shifting from sole attention on the dependence, frailty and poor health of older people towards healthy and productive ageing.

AGEING IN RURAL AND REMOTE COMMUNITIES

Within Australia, the growing ageing population is nowhere more evident than in rural and regional locations. Here, the population is ageing disproportionately, as well over a third of older people (aged over 65 years) live outside major Australian cities and this number is increasing steadily (AIHW, 2007). This is a result of two concurrent trends: older people are remaining in rural areas as the young move away in search of employment and education, while at the same time older people are actively moving to rural areas as tree-changers, seeking a rural lifestyle and cheaper housing.

Yet ageing in rural areas can be problematic, as rural communities often comprise some of the most disadvantaged and socially excluded parts of Australia (Alston, 2005b). Older people in rural areas are vulnerable to both the disadvantages associated with rural living and those associated with ageing (Winterton & Warburton, 2010). These include economic disadvantages, such as low incomes, and health and social disadvantages associated with geographic isolation. These disadvantages have been identified as a key challenge to healthy ageing in Australia (Davis & Bartlett, 2008).

One of the major disadvantages associated with ageing in a rural area is the shortage of health and aged care services, which makes it difficult to access good health care. There are clearly problems in delivering services effectively and efficiently in a geographically dispersed area. Many rural communities struggle to access health services, with associated difficulties in recruiting and retaining a health and aged care workforce (Winterton & Warburton, 2010). Services are costly to provide in rural communities, yet the alternative is for older people to travel to regional centres to visit hospital or specialist health services. Some home and community care workers provide important outreach services, which involve many hours of travelling to visit one or two clients living in geographically isolated locations. As a result, rural older people have higher morbidity and mortality rates, despite the image of a healthy outdoor lifestyle (Alston, 2004b).

As well as disadvantages, however, there is also evidence of some positive aspects of rural ageing. The literature highlights the potential benefits of a healthy, active rural lifestyle, particularly noting the strong sense of community often said to exist in small rural communities (Winterton & Warburton, 2010). This literature suggests that high levels of social capital in rural areas can compensate for some of the disadvantages associated with rural ageing. In particular, social capital can counter social isolation and loneliness, mitigate against some of the losses associated with ageing, and as a result improve individual health outcomes. A recent study of social capital in a rural area found older groups had significant close relationships with friends and neighbours, and were involved in service clubs, church groups, neighbourhood groups and local politics (Hodgkin, 2010). In social work practice, it is important that this not be overlooked, as the majority of older Australians enjoy small but rich networks of social support provided by their communities.

In rural and remote communities, the potential for exclusion also needs to be considered. This can be due to geographic isolation, living out of town, or having transport and access difficulties. Social capital also needs to be considered carefully, as Karen Healy and Anne Hampshire (2002) suggest, as it can have a 'dark side' associated with exclusionary processes or it can mask other forms of disadvantage. A focus on generating social capital can also lead to governments opting out in favour of community-run programs. The success of such programs in generating new social capital has yet to be empirically proven.

LIVELIHOOD AND RETIREMENT

The concept of rurality is important, as it determines the ways in which older people think about their identity and their everyday lives, and this is particularly true for those who both live and work on the land (Thompson & Gullifer, 2006). As discussed in Chapter 1, the social construction of farming leads to some key narratives or themes such as toughness, a down-to-earth worldview, attachment to place and the importance of continuing to feel productive and useful as farmers age (Thompson & Gullifer, 2006). Farming is more than a way of life and provides a strong cultural identity for many Australians, in a large country where 60 per cent of the continent is used for agriculture or grazing (Australian Government, 2007).

Yet rural Australia is in the midst of a period of significant structural change as a result of uncertain economic and climatic conditions such as globalisation and drought (Australian Government, 2007). This has seen the decline and often failure of small to middle-sized farms and the growth of large farm business enterprises. Despite this growth, Australian agriculture is still dominated by farm families, with nearly all broad acre and dairy farms operating as family farms (Alston, 2004b). Farming in Australia has traditionally been undertaken by families as a business passed on to successive generations. While there is some decline in the overall numbers of farm families, they still dominate the agricultural sector. However, in the face of drought and economic problems, many of these families are becoming increasingly dependent on off-farm employment to maintain an income, with Alston (2004b) noting that half of farm families rely on off-farm income to ensure that they can remain in farming. Much of this off-farm work is undertaken by women, placing severe strains on family networks.

Farming is increasingly becoming an ageing phenomenon, particularly as fewer young people are choosing agriculture for their future. Since the mid-1970s, the number of young people entering farming has more than halved as a result of poor returns, the difficulties of working in a family environment and the perceptions of greater opportunities elsewhere (Barr et al., 2005). Young farmers are also aware of the difficulties of maintaining a social life and finding a partner, perhaps epitomised in the TV show *The Farmer Wants a Wife*. As a result, the median age of the farming population has increased and many farming families are ageing without any clear options for the future.

The National Farmers' Federation's 2008 Labour Shortage Action Plan has identified that there are now fewer young people working on farms, leading to farmers having to work for longer. The end result is that farmers are ageing far more rapidly than other groups of workers, with a quarter of farm owners aged 65 years and over compared with only 5 per cent of owner-managers in other industry sectors (Foskey, 2005; Hicks et al., 2008).

These current economic and social circumstances provide multiple challenges for older people who have traditionally lived off the land, particularly in the face of widespread drought and increased rural poverty (Alston, 2004b). Generally, the drought crisis has led to significant personal hardship, requiring a focused social work response in the form of counselling and suicide-prevention groups (Hall & Scheltens, 2005). Further, as a result of these challenges, young people are becoming increasingly reluctant to inherit the property, and older farmers are forced to delay retirement and remain in farming despite of, or because of, poverty (Alston, 2004b). Succession planning becomes a critical issue for many of these families.

SUCCESSION PLANNING

Globalisation and cultural change have led to movements of individuals and populations, and to the breakdown of families located within one geographical area. Nowhere is this more significant than in rural Australia, where farming is traditionally a family affair and properties tend to be passed down through the generations.

Australian agriculture has been impacted significantly over recent decades by globalisation, changes to the market, commodity fluctuations and climatic conditions such as drought (Alston, 2004b). Economic and environmental crises in recent years are leading to stress among farm families, with many living well below the average wage, and increasingly needing welfare and counselling services (Hall & Scheltens, 2005). These occupational burdens continue to fall on farmers who are themselves ageing.

As Daniela Stehlik (2009) notes, the intergenerational arrangements among landowners date back to the Middle Ages. In recent years, there are challenges to the current order whereby maintenance of family living standards are gaining priority over preserving the family's ties with the land. This suggests conflict between two trends—farming as a lifestyle and farming as a business (Barr et al.,

2005). As life expectancy has increased, the transition time lengthens, and in many cases the next generation has left the farm before there is any serious consideration of succession (Stehlik, 2009). Younger family members are then reluctant to return to take over the property, having made a life elsewhere. In turn, many of the older generation are also reluctant to pass on such a problematic business venture to the young. Inheritance becomes extremely problematic, and many older farmers are faced with few options and an unstable future. Thus increasing life expectancy coupled with economic and social change have altered the balance between generations in farming (Foskey, 2005). This highlights the importance of three interrelated processes—retirement, inheritance and succession—which raises some significant issues for rural social work practice.

Retirement is a problematic concept for older farmers. First, with declining farm incomes, many farmers are forced to work on past the age at which others retire (Hicks et al., 2008). Second, while they may wish to move off the property and into the local town, this may be financially impossible with the only alternative being the loss of the farm as an inheritance. Third, there are significant psychological issues associated with retirement as a major life change. This is particularly the case for those such as farmers who have their identity tied up with work, and may be reluctant to retire because of the negative connotations associated with retirement (Foskey, 2005).

Discussions about inheritance and succession present difficult terrain to navigate. In particular, many farmers struggle to maintain a viable business for the next generation, wanting to treat all children fairly as well as provide for their own retirement (Barclay et al., 2007). According to a major government report, most farmers believe that passing the farm on to a sole heir is the best way to maintain the farm within the family and ensure its viability (Barclay et al., 2007). Despite this, research has shown that succession and inheritance are not discussed within farming families, and over 20 per cent of them found farm transfer to be very stressful (Crosby, 1998).

SOCIAL WORK PRACTICE WITH OLDER PEOPLE LIVING IN RURAL AND REMOTE AREAS

This backdrop of social issues highlights the complexities older Australians face living in rural and remote areas. Despite these concerns, it appears that social work practice in this area is fairly limited, and the needs of farm families are not well understood. In order to work effectively, social workers need to develop an under-standing of the complexity of retirement and succession planning issues, along with the complex intergenerational tensions associated with farming life.

Social workers can play a critical role in helping families move away from understanding ageing as loss and decline towards under-standing change in relation to life stage theory and adaptation. The life course perspective, familiar to social work, draws on a range of theoretical perspectives to understand major life transitions. This perspective offers social workers ways to assess major life course issues, and signal the skills and supports needed to adapt to change. In particular, the adoption of strength-based approaches—identifying areas of resilience, coping and support—remains salient in working with older people.

Ageing is shaped by a combination of biological, psychological and social developments (Greene, 2008). Roberta R. Greene has devel-oped the Functional Age Assessment Tool to enable social workers to better identify the multifaceted and interrelated factors directly related to life course adaptation. Using the tool, social workers can address the physiological aspects of ageing. As noted earlier, a quarter of all farmers are aged 65 and over, and although farming remains hard physical work, many of these older farmers cannot afford to retire. While there is recognition that there is considerable variability in physical ageing and its impact on work patterns and health, how individuals adapt to physiological change remains important for social workers to assess. In this regard, Margret M. Baltes and Laura L. Carstensen's (1996) model of successful adaptation to ageing is useful for social work practice. These authors propose a theory that promotes minimisation of loss and maximisation of gain through three strategies. The first of these strategies involves *selection*—either increasing or limiting the number of activities performed in anticipa-tion of change. Selection may involve making environmental changes, and in the case of an ageing farmer may ultimately mean selling the farm and relocating or beginning family discussions about succession planning. The second strategy, *compensation*, involves promoting the use of aids, including memory and technological aids, in order to maximise functioning. Here the ageing farmer may look at hiring additional help to minimise the physical aspects of the work. The third strategy, *optimisation*, involves the promotion of behaviours that enhance functioning and adaptive fitness. Here it is important to select activities that bring satisfaction and enjoyment. A social work practitioner might use this model to discuss someone's desired goals and the processes required to achieve them.

Social work can also play a vital role in addressing the practical and financial issues associated with ageing and retirement. In terms of retirement, Roslyn Foskey (2005), for example, suggests that there is a strong need for retirement planning education programs. She also suggests that a focus on retirement as a concept can be difficult as it may be viewed as an ending—particularly associated with giving up farming—rather than seen as the beginning of a new stage of life (Foskey, 2005). This is an important role for retirement planning: to extend into a whole-of-life approach, and to build positive mental health approaches. Many ageing farmers now need to draw on welfare assistance but there may be little discussion about financial issues within the family (Hicks et al., 2008). In this context, practitioners can play a role in facilitating such discussions within the family.

By adopting a life course perspective, the transitions and experiences of individuals are very closely linked to other family members across generations. Thus social work with older people frequently involves using an intergenerational approach. The need for succession planning, identified earlier in this chapter, further complicates intergenerational relationships with issues of obligation, responsibility and inheritance rarely being discussed. Any work with older rural Australians needs to encompass an understanding of each family member's perspective across the generations. Practitioners should also be mindful of the variability of intergenerational relationships. For instance, some may be quite strong, with high levels of emotional closeness and mutual support. Other family relationships may be characterised by a sense of obligation where high levels of structural connectedness are evident yet only average levels of functional exchange exist. Some families may be characterised by high levels of conflict, low solidarity and intergenerational ambivalence (Silverstein & Bengston, 1997). New roles and changes in decision-making are likely to be negotiated among family members at times when retirement and succession planning are being considered.

Working from an intergenerational approach, Elizabeth Anne Curtis and Marion Shirley Dixon (2005) discuss the importance of mapping roles, relationships and beliefs through each generation. They also suggest distinguishing between situational difficulties, such as dealing with a medical crisis, and unresolved transitions or chronic relationship difficulties. These authors argue that this distinction between different factors creating change will subsequently influence the method of intervention. For instance, with situational difficulties the intervention might focus on the provision of support and education. With transition and chronic relationship difficulties, there is an opportunity to address long-standing tensions through family counselling.

In relation to social work with older people, it is equally important to develop an assessment of the community, understanding the complex informal networks that provide varying levels of support to those living in rural and remote areas. There has been extensive research that examines the social networks of older people. This research has identified the importance of a small but close network of friends and neighbours providing reciprocal support and assistance (Kendig, 2000), with knowledge and assessment of social supports beyond the family being particularly important in rural and remote areas.

Practitioners working with older people in rural and remote areas must also deal with significant practical dilemmas. Earlier in the chapter, the shortage of health and aged care services was noted. There is also a scarcity of aged care specialists. Access to such limited service delivery is complicated by distance and the availability of public transportation. These limitations make comprehensive assessment more problematic. Future advances in technology are viewed as a solution to combating geographical isolation. Angela Crombie and colleagues (2009) contend that recent advances in telecommunication technologies are increasing access to health services for people living in rural and remote areas. Here the introduction of tele-health and related services such as tele-psychiatry, tele-rehabilitation and tele-cardiology can be used to facilitate both the exchange of health information and the provision of health-care services. Crombie et al. (2009) argue that current and future rural health-care workers will be required to be abreast of advances in technology. How successful such technologies will be in the delivery of services in working with older people in rural and remote areas has yet to be empirically tested. However, social work practitioners working in rural and remote areas increasingly will have access to technologies such as video conferencing to assist in making assessments.

CASE STUDY: KEN AND MARGARET

Ken is a 69-year-old man who lives with his wife, Margaret, on their cattle farm in central New South Wales. Ken had worked the farm with his father since leaving high school. His father passed away some time ago. Ken and Margaret continue to provide care for his mother, Ruby (aged 89). Margaret now believes Ruby's care needs have become too difficult for her to manage. They have recently discussed the option of moving Ruby to a high-care facility, in a regional city 30 kilometres from the farm.

Ken and Margaret had hoped to retire late in their sixties and move into the regional city to be closer to Ruby, and to their children and grandchildren. Ken and Margaret have two children, Tom (aged 44) and Catherine (aged 42). They have four grandchildren. They had envisaged passing the property on to Tom; however, he has shown little interest in farming.

The farm has been struggling financially. They have limited investment funds set aside to support their retirement, and have been told it is unlikely that they would be successful in selling their farm for the price they had hoped. They had anticipated being able to invest from the sale of the farm. They have been talking with a rural financial counsellor, and recently with the bank manager, about the property's increasing debt level. The ongoing drought has meant they have had to reduce the size of their herd, and face ongoing problems with providing sufficient water and feed.

Ken suffers chronic back pain from a previous farm injury, which has severely restricted his mobility. Margaret has ongoing pain from arthritis. Their children have become concerned about both Ken and Margaret's ability to manage the farm. On a recent visit home, Catherine spoke with a local drought support worker. This worker told Catherine that he too has become concerned about Ken's ability to cope with his property, and has visited Ken and Margaret a number of times due to problems with his stock and pasture management. When Catherine pressed Margaret, she confessed that she thought the farm was 'too much for them now', but feels she can't talk to Ken about this. Margaret has become extremely worried about Ken's emotional state. He is drinking more than usual, and appears to have lost interest in the property and his usual social activities. Margaret is also worried about Ruby, and how she will cope with moving into the high-care facility.

Catherine spoke with Tom and they agreed that the best option was for Ken and Margaret to sell the property, regardless of the financial consequences. Catherine has organised for the family to discuss this transition with a social worker at the local Community Health Centre.

Reflections

- Prepare an initial assessment of Ken and Margaret. In doing so, identify the micro, meso and macro issues impacting the family.
- Using an intergenerational method of practice, highlight the issues facing each family member. Role-play with each family member to develop these issues further.
- Plan a family meeting that will include all members of the family. What issues would you consider important to discuss in such a meeting? What skills would you be drawing upon? Role-play the family meeting.

SUMMARY

This chapter has focused on the key issues encountered by older people living in rural and remote areas of Australia and examined the current challenges facing farming families, whose livelihoods have been impacted by globalisation, climate change and drought. A range of complex issues facing older farming families, including loss of farm income leading to a delay in retirement age, and intergenerational issues involved in succession planning, have been highlighted. In presenting these issues, it is argued that social work practice in this area is limited and the needs of farming families have not been addressed sufficiently. A focus on life course and intergenerational relationships, taking into account the biological, psychological and social aspects of ageing, is proposed as a way forward.

RECOMMENDED READING

Alston, M. (2004) Social capital in rural Australia. *Rural Society*, 12(2), 93–104.

Davis, S. & Bartlett, H. (2008) Healthy ageing in rural Australia: Issues and challenges. *Australasian Journal on Ageing*, 27(2), 56–60.

Hughes, M. & Heycox, K. (2010) *Older People, Ageing and Social Work*. Allen & Unwin, Sydney.

Naughtin, G. & Schofield, V. (2009) Working with older people. In M. Connolly & L. Harms (eds), *Social Work, Contexts and Practice*. Oxford University Press, Melbourne, pp. 195–208.

14

ADDRESSING THE EFFECTS OF CLIMATE CHANGE ON RURAL COMMUNITIES

Margaret Alston

CHAPTER OBJECTIVES

- To provide an outline of the concepts of climate change and gender.
- To examine social and demographic changes occurring in rural inland Australia.
- To outline the impacts of climate change in these regions.
- To provide an understanding of the adaptations of individuals and families, particularly farming families.
- To develop an understanding of the service infrastructure in inland areas.
- To analyse policy and service elements that shape or restrict positive and sustainable adaptations.
- To provide an introduction to a sustainable development framework.
- To present details of a model of social work service provision that will aid the sustainable development of the inland regions of Australia.

INTRODUCTION

Regardless of the likely impacts of any fundamental changes in climate, inland areas of Australia have been undergoing significant restructuring for at least the last 50 years. This restructuring, which has changed the face of rural Australia, results from wide-ranging phenomena such as globalisation; declining employment; population outmigration as people drift to the cities and coast in search of jobs, education or a better lifestyle; the loss of services and infrastructure; free trade agreements, which have often reduced prices for agricultural products and therefore rural prosperity; and the declining political influence of the rural constituency. Overlaid on these factors in recent times has been the impact of climate events—both incremental, such as drought, and catastrophic, such as bushfires and floods—which have exacerbated the reshaping of rural areas.

The drought has been a feature of inland agricultural regions for over a decade, leaving families and businesses in crisis, communities depleted and the landscapes surrounding these areas shattered. Meanwhile, a number of catastrophic events—such as the Victorian bushfires and floods in northern New South Wales and Queensland—have also created sudden and destructive change in many small inland communities. These events have had an equally devastating effect on people, communities and landscape. Yet there has been a serious lack of political attention to the social impacts of climate change, with few community services in these areas addressing climate change management and a noticeable lack of social workers and other health professionals working with people to adapt in positive ways to major changes. Arguably, this is a result of a number of factors related to the principles underpinning policy formulation and service provision. However, it also results from our failure to recognise the *environment* as an emerging field of social work practice and a domain where social workers can provide leadership by focusing attention on a more sustainable development framework and therefore a more satisfying quality of life.

Beginning with an explanation of the key concepts of climate change and gender, this chapter outlines the impacts of climate change in rural and remote inland areas, and examines the resultant gendered social impacts. It also details service infrastructure and other policy initiatives designed to address climate events, but which largely neglect the social impacts or address either the increasing vulnerability of people of the inland or the social fragmentation in rural communities. The chapter addresses the complex notion that adaptations to climate change have been highly gendered and not always positive, and that if we are to foster sustainable adaptations and build resilience in these communities, gender must be acknowledged as a significant variable in how people adapt. Finally, the chapter outlines a model of practice and service innovation that will assist these inland regions to develop in more creative ways, and at the same time provide satisfying work experiences for human service personnel.

CLIMATE CHANGE

Climate change results from a build-up of greenhouse gases in the atmosphere as a result of the burning of fossil fuels and deforestation (McMichael, 2003); these have increased by over 70 per cent since 1970 (IPCC, 2007). This build-up results in melting of the polar ice caps, rising temperatures and sea levels, changing weather patterns (producing droughts) and extreme weather events (such as fires, floods and tsunamis) (IPCC, 2007). While the scientific community is largely of the view that climate change is human-made, there is still scepticism in the community as to the causes and permanency of climate change—though there is general agreement that world food and water security is under threat.

For communities and people reliant on agriculture as their main industry and employment base, drought and unusual weather events have created high levels of uncertainty, and further destabilised regions already undergoing significant restructuring. Areas like the Murray-Darling Basin—the food bowl of Australia—which relies on irrigated agriculture for products such as citrus fruits, grapes, dairy and vegetable production, are heavily impacted by the reduced water available to produce food. Farmers and businesses reliant on agri-cultural production are unsure about whether to continue to farm in areas that are becoming increasingly unviable. As the drought has dragged on, and catastrophic events such as fires and floods are occurring with alarming regularity, the spectre of irreversible climate change has become a very real feature of life in inland regions.

Nonetheless, there are many sceptics who dispute the idea of irre-versible climate change or its causes, and a large proportion of the population of inland Australia is among them. This is understandable, as the alternative threatens the traditional rural way of life. Regard-less of the permanency of climate change or its causes, it is evident that the climate variability of the past decade has had major impacts on the lives of people in rural and remote areas, that these impacts have exacerbated and accelerated change in these inland regions, that social policy has failed to address adequately the social disintegration occurring in many of these small communities, and that the ability of people and communities to positively adapt in sustainable ways is therefore limited.

Australia is not alone in its experiences of climate variability and extreme weather events. Globally, it is impossible to understand the significance of climate change without a contextual understanding of the world population explosion and increasing global poverty. Population on our planet is predicted to rise from six to nine billion by 2050, further—and critically—exacerbating food and water insecurity. As Abigail Jones and colleagues (2009: 10) note:

> Around the world, extreme poverty fuels a volatile mix of desperation and instability—exhausting governing institutions, depleting resources, weakening leaders and crushing hope.

This volatile mix of poverty, rising numbers of people on the planet, climate variability and extreme weather events is causing major problems across the world. Yet the urgent need to address and reduce greenhouse gas emissions in order to reduce the threat of climate instability is creating major global political tensions.

In an attempt to address climate change, the United Nations Framework Convention on Climate Change (UNFCC) was adopted in 1997 and nations were urged to sign up to reduce greenhouse gas emissions in what has become known as the Kyoto Protocol. The Australian government under John Howard refused to sign, but the first act of the Rudd Labor government elected in 2007 was to sign the Protocol. Despite being widely supported, the United Nations Climate Change Conference held in Copenhagen, Denmark, in 2009 and attended by 120 heads of governments failed to achieve its goal of a binding agreement on the reduction of global greenhouse gas emissions. Conflicts occurred between developed and developing nations, and there was reluctance from countries such as the United States and Australia to adopt significant reduction targets. These negotiations are far removed from the everyday experiences of families experiencing the daily reality of climate change/variability.

There is major disquiet in the scientific community about the failure of global leaders to act decisively on climate change, and predictions have been made that a crisis is looming (Hamilton, 2010; Garnaut, 2008). There is also some suggestion that a failure on the part of former Australian prime minister Kevin Rudd to act more decisively on climate measures was a factor in his loss of the prime ministership to Julia Gillard in June 2010. There is no doubt that climate change is a politically charged topic, that there is still insufficient action around climate change-mitigation strategies across the world, and that it will lead to a decreasing ability to address global food and water security. Critically, the IPCC is predicting that the twenty-first century will be dominated by resource wars (Giddens, 2009) and commentators such as Maude Barlow (2007) predict that a lack of access to fresh water will lead to significant global destabilisation.

In Australia, we are already experiencing conflict relating to water access as declining water stocks pit environmentalists against irrigation farmers, and city populations against rural townships. Australia is one of the driest continents on the planet, and our experiences of hotter temperatures and more unpredictable weather over the last decade have left us with reduced water availability and reduced capacity for food production. Those living in inland Australia are at the coalface of climate change events, yet they have limited resources with which to deal with these major uncertainties. For the most part, they are impoverished farm families and rural residents. Yet the politically charged context in which discussions of climate change take place does little to address with any degree of integrity the circumstances or uncertainties facing these families and communities. Before we examine the social and demographic features of rural Australia and the gendered adaptations occurring in these areas, a brief definition of what is meant by gender is provided in order to understand how it is possible that the women and men of inland Australia might experience climate change/variability differently.

GENDER

Quite apart from biological differences between men and women, gender refers to the way we operate in the world as masculine or feminine, filtered by the constraints of social norms and practices, and aided by institutions such as the church, the law and the family. Women are more constrained by these normative processes and, because they represent up to 70 per cent of the world's poor (CBD, UNEP & IUCN, 2007), are more vulnerable to climate change impacts. For example, Eric Neumayer and Thomas Pluemper's (2007) research suggests that women are up to fourteen times more likely to die in natural disasters. In Australia, as in the rest of the world, women are less likely to own land and resources needed for food production, and as water becomes a valuable tradable commodity, they are less likely to own and control this precious resource. In Australia, water licences are more likely to be owned by men, making women particularly vulnerable to changes in water regulation and community access to water.

Women are particularly vulnerable to gender-based inequalities, yet are far less likely to be represented in forums where decisions relating to climate change are made. Thus there is increasing recognition that climate change will have variable gendered impacts (FAO, 2007; Alber, 2011) and that poor rural women in particular will be most severely impacted (Alber, 2011). Before discussing the gendered impacts of climate change in Australia, an understanding of the social and demographic factors evident in our rural inland areas will give an idea of the increasing vulnerability of rural populations.

CLIMATE CHANGE IMPACTS ON A VULNERABLE POPULATION

The climate events outlined above—the drought and extreme weather events—have exposed already-vulnerable rural people to increasing uncertainty. Agricultural production has been affected significantly by drought, and water shortages have resulted in irrigation farmers being denied access to water, further reducing their income-producing capacity. Over several years, the writer has undertaken research in the vast inland areas of rural Australia and seen at first hand the impacts of ongoing climate change. Population drift has accelerated, particularly from the more remote areas; health impacts have been exacerbated; mental health impacts are very evident; relationships problems are increasing; service support is decreasing.

In areas where extreme weather events have taken place, the disaster-recovery process is one of heightened stress, likely loss of property and possessions, tension within families, and uncertainty about rebuilding lives in familiar places or moving to start a new life elsewhere. For those living at the edge of the climate change experience, quality of life has eroded at a time when supports and services that may have aided more positive adaptations have declined.

It is also evident that the impacts of these changes are highly gendered. Drought, for example, highlights the differing gendered experiences of climate events. Because women and men come to agriculture through different pathways, their experiences of drought and level of influence relating to agricultural production and policy vary.

Men are far more likely to inherit agricultural land and women are more likely to come to agriculture through marriage. Men are more likely to undertake the physically demanding tasks associated with agricultural production, while women are more likely to have higher educational qualifications, to undertake farm financial management and to be working off the farm. These differing work experiences lead also to differential experiences of climate change. For farm men, their physical work leads them to work daily in barren landscapes, undertaking the repetitive tasks of hand-feeding and watering live-stock. Women are more likely to be aware of the financial position of the enterprise, to be exposed to the vagaries of the rural labour market and to the lack of services such as child care. Research also exposes the gendered experiences of dramatic events such as bush-fires and post-disaster recovery (Proudley, 2008). Thus the ways in which women and men adapt to these stressful circumstances are also likely to differ.

CLIMATE CHANGE ADAPTATIONS

Adaptation refers to the ways in which people and communities respond to the pressures they are experiencing. It is highly dependent on the resilience or capacity of people and communities to respond effectively. Adaptations to dramatic events can be positive, enabling sustainable change, or negative, resulting in unsustainable adjust-ments; it is often dependent on the level of individual and community resilience. The resilience of rural people and communities has been eroded over a number of years as a result of unpredictable climate changes. John W. Handmer and Stephen R. Dovers (2009) note that resilience can be reactive—that is, where people and communi-ties resist change and seek to operate as they have always done—or it can be proactive: that is, where people and communities accept that change is inevitable and work to adapt in positive and sustain-able ways. Reactive resilience—and therefore unsustainable adjust-ments—appears to be dominant in rural inland areas because of the long years of drought, but also the lack of informed policy and a dearth of services and support.

Further, gendered adaptations are evident in research conducted with farm family members coping with drought. For example, men often report that they long for a return to 'normality', or a more traditional lifestyle, while women are more likely to report that they are ready to leave for a new life (Alston et al., under review). Many families are taking on increased levels of debt as they attempt to stay in farming, further adding to the anxieties and stresses of farming. They also report health impacts, including extraordinary stress and a stoicism that makes them resistant to seeking help (Alston, 2010). As a result, it is evident that a high-priority adaptation among farm families is the sourcing of off-farm income, and this is most often undertaken by women. A majority of farm women of working age are in the paid workforce, and our research confirms that there are significant stresses associated with long-distance travel to work, a lack of child care and, for many, the need to live away from home in order to find work. Women report that the juggling of workloads creates significant stress and a need to spread themselves across a number of areas in order to assist and support all members of the family (Alston et al., under review). Both men and women report relationship tensions and health issues, and both see an uncertain future for farm families. Higher levels of domestic violence in these areas are further evidence of gendered reactions to these pressures.

These more reactive adaptations are exacerbated by the uncertainty of the political response to climate change. Many rural people report that they feel demonised as environmental vandals by the Australian community because food production is resource intensive. They also report feeling alienated from the rest of the population, and outside the political decision-making processes so crucial to their continued viability. Climate change/variability is having a significant impact on people in inland Australia, and yet the social policy response has been limited. One result is a lack of attention to the need to develop a sustainable regional response, one that supports people and communities at the forefront of climate impacts.

POLICY AND SERVICES THAT AID OR RESTRICT SUSTAINABLE ADAPTATIONS

Over a number of years, governments of all persuasions have adopted a neo-liberal philosophy in relation to services and infrastructure. This philosophy dictates that government withdraw from the front line of service provision, preferring instead to privatise welfare service delivery by funding civil society organisations to deliver services. These organisations are often underfunded and employ people on short-term contracts and with restricted employment conditions. In inland areas, these services may reduce costs by employing welfare workers rather than social workers, and overusing volunteers at the front line of service delivery. At the same time, many services have adopted a user-pays system to increase funds available for service support. Hubs of centralised service have developed in regional centres and capital cities as government service infrastructure is centralised and regionalised.

Thus the neo-liberal policy framework has resulted in processes of privatisation, marketisation (Healy & Meagher, 2000), regionalisation and centralisation, which have produced an ad hoc and unplanned service infrastructure in many smaller communities. Some communities are overserviced in some areas and underserviced in others. The result is a lack of certainty around service support for people in small communities despite their increased vulnerability.

There has also been a shift in policy emphasis from a community-minded approach to an expectation on the part of governments that people should look after themselves or that care needs should be absorbed within the family. This has impacted rural families in various ways, particularly as rural women are now working in similar proportions to their urban counterparts. Their experiences of workforce participation are more fraught, however, because of a lack of child care, aged care and disability care, and work conditions that may be inflexible and family unfriendly.

A further example of policy failure relates to the difficulties experienced by impoverished farm families in crisis attempting to access household income support. Farming families are not eligible for unemployment benefits but may access Exceptional Circumstances payments for household income support. However, the difficulties associated with eligibility have resulted in fewer than 20 per cent of farm families accessing payments at any one time despite the drought, lack of income and high levels of debt (Alston & Kent, 2006). As a result, farm poverty has become a significant feature of rural life.

Water policy is another example of a climate change mitigation policy that pays scant regard to social outcomes. This policy is based on economic and environmental outcomes, and has resulted in significant anxiety and stress for families and communities reliant on irrigated agriculture.

In summary, while processes of change and restructuring have been evident in rural inland areas for decades, climate change/ variability has exacerbated and accelerated these processes. At the same time, isolation and a lack of access to suitable services have resulted in evident disadvantage among rural populations on a number of indicators, including health, welfare, education and employment.

Policies and programs have exacerbated socio-economic disadvantage, reducing the ability of people to adapt to climate change and ongoing restructuring in proactive ways. Resilience in rural areas has been reduced by a lack of government attention, as well as a policy framework that is largely dismissive of social outcomes, is individualistic and does little to build resilience or positive adaptation. A more viable solution to inland community crises lies in generating a sustainable development framework.

SUSTAINABLE DEVELOPMENT FRAMEWORK

The concept of sustainable development emerged from the World Commission on Environment and Development's Brundtland Report of 1987. This report defined sustainable development as 'a development that meets the needs of the present without compromising the ability of future generations to meet their own needs' (WCED, 1987: 46).

A sustainable development framework incorporates not only environmental and economic security, but must have as its basis the concept of social sustainability. Social sustainability is defined as the 'capacity of a society to provide for the wellbeing of its people in an equitable manner' (Tonts, 2005: 199). Incorporating economic, environmental and social sustainability into a definition of a sustainable rural community, Alan Black (2005: 27) describes such a community as one where:

- the environment sustains humans and other species
- the economy adapts to change, provides long-term security to residents and recognises environmental limitations, and
- the community provides a social foundation for the health of all residents, respecting cultural diversity, equity and the needs of future generations.

The idea of sustainable rural development has gained currency in the rest of the world. For example, the European Conference on Rural Development held in Ireland in 1996 produced the Cork Declaration, which notes in part that

> sustainable rural development must be put at the top of the agenda of the European Union . . . [and that this] aims to reduce out-migration, combat poverty, stimulate employment and equality of opportunity,

and respond to growing requests for more quality health, safety, personal development and leisure and improved rural wellbeing. (European Commission, 1996)

Sustainable rural development should also acknowledge the gendered experiences of women and men, as well as the need to be gender-sensitive in programmatic responses.

It is evident that Australia is far from considering a sustainability framework. The commitment to a market-based approach and the lack of a concerted voice of representation for rural people have led to an arrogant and benign institutional neglect of rural people and places (Molnar, 2010). With the ongoing changes being experienced by vulnerable rural populations, it is timely for Australia to pay greater attention to a sustainable development framework, one that attends as much to the social as it does to the economic and environmental. It is the writer's contention in this chapter that social workers are in an ideal position to address this shortcoming.

SOCIAL WORK SERVICE PROVISION FOR SUSTAINABLE DEVELOPMENT

Critical problems in attracting social workers to rural areas include a lack of supervision and the difficulties associated with working in isolation. Addressing these issues is essential to a successful model of social work service to isolated areas. Elsewhere, the writer has argued for a model of rural service provision based on a sustainable development framework with social workers as critical players in developing and adapting the model (Alston, 2009a). In summary, the role of social workers would include understanding and recording the needs of rural communities and people, advocating for government attention to these needs, arguing for governments to move away from a market-based approach to service provision, and developing an Australian sustainability framework.

To overcome identified problems, a model of service provision into stressed inland communities affected by significant social change might include the use of regional service hubs to employ and supervise community development social workers, who would spend half of their time in their allocated rural community undertaking community development work, building networks, forming inter-agency councils, assisting communities to develop plans and grant applications and developing inclusive, gender-sensitive sustainability projects. Back at their regional hubs, social workers could work with their supervisors to refine plans and applications, network and advocate with governments and NGOs, and work with other community development workers to develop new ideas and programs and to extend the sustainability framework to incorporate identified issues. A big part of their role would be to lobby governments on behalf of their rural constituents, and to bring to government and community attention the issues and challenges facing rural people challenged by climate change and resultant gendered social impacts.

Social workers would work with governments and communities to develop sustainable adaptations to climate events and to reframe rural communities as viable and attractive places to live. Social workers are ideally placed to develop a sustainable development framework for rural inland Australia that is socially inclusive, responsive and innovative. Working with communities at the nexus of policy and people, social workers have the skills to formulate a more enduring model of rural sustainability, one that values people over profits.

CASE STUDY: ADVANCING WOMEN FARMERS GRANTS PROGRAM

In 2009 and 2010, the Australian government, through the federal Department of Agriculture, Fisheries and Forests, offered grants of up to $50000 to rural women's groups across Australia to develop women's programs and to enhance the status of women. The program, called Advancing Women Farmers, was highly successful in mobilising rural women to form groups and organise inclusive social events and programs. Most of these grants were given to women in small rural communities, and resulted in a wealth of activity and energetic attention to community adaptations.

The writer was successful in gaining one of these grants to work with rural women to develop an understanding of the impact of climate change on women. The culmination of this work was a forum held in Melbourne in 2009, just prior to the Copenhagen Climate Change Conference. The forum attracted a large, diverse group of rural women from across Australia who wanted a voice in the climate change debate and wished to express their views on the impact of climate change on rural women. Many women reported that this was the first time they had been given a forum in which to highlight the gendered impacts and to voice their concerns about the lack of attention to gender issues, the lack of consultation with women and the failure of policy to address the issues facing women and their families.

This case study highlights, first, the usefulness of offering a small grants program for women only, and second, the responsiveness of women to participating when they are invited to do so. On the negative side, it also highlights the lack of gender-sensitive policy related to climate change and the lack of attention by government to the issues identified by women through this program. The outcomes of the various women's actions undertaken under the Advancing Women Farmers program have not been addressed in any systematic way.

While this was not a social work program, the grant was administered by staff in the Social Work Department at Monash University, and allowed the mobilisation of women around climate change. The small grant scheme indicates that if governments are prepared to offer small amounts of money for rural community development, rural people are highly responsive. It suggests that it may be timely for an approach to government by social work bodies to fund rural community development actions.

FURTHER POSSIBILITIES

In working with the material presented in this chapter, a useful way to connect with the suggested models presented is to locate a small community in your state that has been impacted by a climate change event. Using Australian Bureau of Statistics community profile data, examine the demographic profile of the community. Through government and other websites, determine the climate variation experienced in this community over the last decade. Access a local services directory and determine the type of service infrastructure available in the community. Think about how you would describe the community and its experiences of climate variability over the last decade and analyse whether the services available in the community are such that they provide the support needed by the community to adapt in positive ways. How might a social work response drawing on a sustainable development framework be developed in this community?

RECOMMENDED READING

Alston, M. (2009) *Innovative Human Services Practice: Changing landscapes*. Pan Macmillan, Melbourne.

Mearns, R. & Norton, A. (eds) (2010) *Social Dimensions of Climate Change: Equity and vulnerability in a warming world*. World Bank, Geneva. <http://web.worldbank.org/WBSITE/EXTERNAL/TOPICS/EX TSOCIALDEVELOPMENT/0,,contentMDK:22408501~pagePK:21005 8~piPK:210062~theSitePK:244363,00.html>, viewed 2 February 2011.

PART IV

Future agenda for social work practice

15

RURAL PRACTICE: AN AGENDA FOR THE FUTURE

Jane Maidment and Uschi Bay

INTRODUCTION

The life course and landscape of rural Australia has been shaped by a diverse array of significant events. The catastrophic impact of European colonisation, the subsequent discovery of gold and other precious minerals, the development of new technologies, and the ongoing emergence of social movements such as feminism and environmentalism have all claimed space and agency in disturbing dominant social, political and economic discourses in rural regions. Observing these major historical influences serves to reinforce that for social work to remain relevant we must critically engage with and be proactive in addressing the ever-changing conditions of those living in rural areas. This level of engagement requires practitioners to focus on working simultaneously in both the micro and macro spheres. Now more than ever, there is an urgency for rural practitioners to perform the tasks of community development, public advocacy and research, along with those roles more traditionally associated with social work practice such as case management, brokerage and counselling.

This analysis of contemporary practice has prompted us to consider how rural social work might look in the future. A careful examination of the social trends and practice responses put forward by contributing authors has enabled us to synthesise five key principles for rural social work practice. We think these principles may in a small way act as a touchstone for future rural social work education, policy, practice and research.

KEY PRINCIPLES FOR FUTURE RURAL SOCIAL WORK

- Recognising the centrality of geography on human life, beyond the notion of the 'person in environment' towards practice embedded in critical ecology, where notions of place, space, sustainability and identity are considered central to personal, community and global well-being.
- Acknowledging the influence of governmentality on the way rural communities position themselves and are positioned in relation to broader policy discourse. Subsequently, using this analysis to foster transformative social relations through practice, policy and research initiatives.
- Embedding practice within a social justice paradigm where the socially stratified nature of power dimensions is made transparent, with an emphasis on equitable social arrangements and a 'whole-of-community' response.
- Fostering interdependency by crossing methodological and theoretical borders between social work and other disciplines, as well as between professional and lay helpers, clients and workers to address the issues of major concern in rural areas.
- Developing comprehensive practitioner researcher knowledge and skills to enhance community planning and policy advocacy initiatives.

The remainder of this chapter is focused on addressing each of these principles with reference to developing a future agenda for rural social work practice, policy and research.

PLACE, SPACE AND SUSTAINABILITY

One issue arising from the material presented in this book is the challenge to social workers to develop a place-based social work model of practice. A conceptual shift and realignment are required to bring geography, ecology and place into the foreground in working with a 'community as a whole' framework. In this context, 'place' is reconceptualised not as background but as the space of 'lived experience'. A spatial understanding of place can open the way for the relations between how the natural world is defined and constituted within institutional practices and within social work theories to be contested. This is considered necessary for social work to take on the challenge of working with regional, rural and remote communities using the notion of 'people as place' to rethink practice in sustainable ecological, social, economical and political ways.

Zapf (2009) proposes that a place-based social work practice is about 'living well in place'. We propose to conceptualise 'living well in place' as an ongoing relationship of 'people as place' that is dynamic, in process and always becoming. This is not a deterministic view of geography, biology or the environment; rather, context and substance—whether these involve issues of housing, violence, climate change, livelihoods or mental health—are inextricably intertwined and mutually constitutive in specific places. Place means location and also the values, meaning and identity associated with that location. 'Assigning meaning to particular locations may not be a uniform or consensual process; different groups can ascribe different meanings or significance to the same region' (Zapf, 2009: 147). For this reason, local knowledges take on renewed importance when working in rural, regional and remote settlements, and with the various sub-groups living there.

The 'whole-of-community' focus in approaching working in a rural, remote and regional setting means also taking into account the diversity of people who live in these locations. It is important to seek out not only the leaders and identified spokespeople, but also people who are usually not engaged with formal community processes; these people need to be identified and brought into discussions about the future of a settlement. From an anti-oppressive perspective, groups who are not involved in decision-making about the community's workings are often marginalised groups. Groups from an anti-oppressive and empowerment perspective are usually marginalised on the basis of gender, class, race, sexual preference, different abilities or age. A 'whole-of-community' approach is inclusive and deliberately seeks to facilitate broad-based discussions formally and informally around livelihood strategies, service development and natural resource management.

One of the central aspects of 'living well in place' is developing an embedded identification with a location based on a 'detailed knowledge of a place, the capacity for observation, a sense of care and rootedness' (Orr, 1992, cited in Zapf, 2009: 153). Many people have become short-term residents, non-permanent residents, temporary workers in regional, rural and remote settings, and this transitory dynamic can be at odds with place-making and living well in place. At times, in-migration of people from cities dislocates local people or disrupts and changes the character or amenity of rural, coastal and remote places considerably.

The competing demands and contestation about places' natural resources, like minerals, water and land use, are part of the dynamic that needs to be addressed in living well in place. These are challenges that many communities have tackled over the last few decades, such as the sea-change phenomenon impacting on the character and amenity of coastal locations. Some current struggles evident in regional, rural and remote settings are about uranium mining in desert Australia, water use negotiations in the Murray-Darling Basin, the use of old-growth forests in Tasmania and the debate about living in fire-prone areas in Victoria, to mention just a few.

For people to learn to live sustainably requires an understanding that 'humans are part of, and not separate from, the dynamic web of life on Earth' (Reed, 2005, cited in Zapf, 2009: 149). An ecosystems approach to social work puts this understanding at the centre of its framework. The 'people as place' metaphor recognises the mutuality of influence between people and places. The challenge for the future is to develop livelihoods that are sustainable in relation to a finite planet. Livelihood analyses also need to deal with the long-term viability of production and exchange practices in the context of complex institutional, capitalist, industrial and local governance arrangements.

The sustainable 'livelihoods perspective starts with questions about how different people live in different places' (Scoones, 2009: 172). The means by which people combine resources and activities in complex ways to make a living encourage social workers to approach rural, remote and regional settlements focused on understanding 'things from a local perspective', which is a negotiated learning between local people and outsiders (2009: 172). The focus is not only on individuals and social problems, but also on concerns with dynamic ecologies, history, gender and social differentiation and cultural practices. Social workers need to be active in identifying the 'political interests, competing discourses and embedded practices' in specific settlements (2009: 181) without losing sight of the macro structural issues.

In the sustainable livelihoods approach, institutions and policies are considered central because they mediate access to resources for people. Social workers from a critical ecological systems theory perspective are alert to the dominant framings of regional, rural and remote communities, and to the politics of knowledge. The production of such knowledge is always conditioned by values, politics, and institutional histories and commitments—which is well illustrated in relation to housing, mental health, governance of homeland communities, child protection, employment, violence and climate change, to mention just a few of the topics covered in the previous chapters.

The challenge for social workers is to develop a place-based model of social work that examines 'networks, linkages, connections, flows and chains across scales, but remains firmly rooted in place and context' (Scoones, 2009: 189). Critical ecological systems theory and an anti-oppressive and empowerment perspective include exploring the particular forms of globalisation and processes of production and exchange. In Australia, they also mean taking into account historical processes of colonialism, high reliance on skilled in-migration of workers from many different cultures, and the current neo-liberal policies that create both processes of marginalisation and opportunity (2009).

GOVERNMENTALITY

The broad definition of government based on Foucault's theorising and used by others like Peter Miller and Nikolas Rose (2008: 27) indicates that a diverse number of groups are seeking 'to regulate the lives of individuals and the conditions within particular national territories in pursuit of various goals'. To think about regional, rural and remote livelihoods through a governmentality perspective means identifying how experts and governments are 'representing' the locality and the issues challenging or confronting the people dwelling there.

In this broader sense, 'government' is always dependent on knowledge of that which is to be governed. There are various ways in which problems are identified, represented, analysed and evaluated by different actors. This knowledge-creation process is always already constitutive of the reality and the people to be acted upon. Political rationalities are the kind of intellectual tools that render 'reality thinkable in such a way that it is amenable to political deliberation' (Miller & Rose, 2008: 59).

In this book, we have indicated a number of ways in which government policy and decision-making at the centre have impacted on regional, rural and remote people and their livelihoods—for instance, in desert homelands, resource boom towns and small agriculturally based towns. A governmentality approach can be used to understand how mechanisms like calculations in one place affect things in another place. One recent example from the Northern Territory Intervention was that local shopkeepers needed to calculate

Aboriginal people's spending to enable central federal government to quarantine and regulate half of each Aboriginal person's Centrelink payments. These calculations are a form of governmental action at a distance. In this way, Centrelink pension recipients can be acted upon and storekeepers enrolled at a distance, in time and space, for the pursuit of social, political and economic policy objectives set at the centre.

Current modes of government often rely on inscription itself as a form of action at a distance. Often governance processes—even in relation to basic service development—demand the collection and aggregation of comprehensive data over various periods of time. Some regional, rural and remote communities are at a marked disadvantage in relation to this kind of data collection. The aggregation of the data itself engages various groups of experts, and requires compliance with the norms and processes of the tender or submission specifications. Through these submission processes, it becomes 'possible to act on events, places and people that are unfamiliar and a long way away', especially if people are dependent upon government funds (Miller & Rose, 2008: 33–4). From a critical ecological systems perspective, social workers are often aware of the simultaneously controlling and enabling aspects of these requirements. Social workers can name and articulate the way these mechanisms operate governmentally to facilitate formal and informal discussions with community members, with the aim of enabling communities to retain some measure of self-determination and say in their destiny.

NEO-LIBERALISM AND 'COMMUNITIES'

Neo-liberalism has informed most policy areas in Australia for the last two decades, and has broadly been concerned with rearranging the relationships between the state, market and communities. In particular, markets were to replace state planning as regulators of economic activity. Within neo-liberal policy regions, rural towns and remote settlements are positioned as economic entrepreneurs in competition with all other places for economic investment and the disinvestment of troublesome populations. Individuals and people living in particular places are positioned 'as active agents seeking to maximize their own advantage [and considered] both the legitimate locus of decisions about their own affairs and the most effective in calculating actions to outcomes' (Miller & Rose, 2008: 79). Regional and rural settings are to promote themselves as offering particular amenities in the global marketplace, and seek to attract investment of all kinds to boost economic productivity and their settlement's economic viability.

Until recently, most attention was focused on how neo-liberalism had informed government relations between the state and markets. However, another equally important consideration relates to the complex way in which 'community' has become surprisingly salient in neo-liberal policy-making. A whole series of issues has been problematised in terms of the features of 'communities', their strengths, cultures and pathologies (Miller & Rose, 2008: 88). There is a whole new territorial imagery of community that shapes the strategies and approaches to issues—for instance, the notion of 'community mental health' (Miller & Rose, 2008: 88). Communities have become 'zones to be investigated, mapped, documented' and programmed through community development programs and community development workers (2008: 88). In Chapter 9, David McCallum outlines how the new child protection policy framework aims to engage 'community' in such a way that it becomes responsible for child protection and for resolving child safety issues.

This trend is evident in the way 'community' was problematised in the Northern Territory Intervention, where Aboriginal individuals were understood as 'subjects of allegiance to a particular set of community values, beliefs and commitments'. This focused the various strategies and programs associated with the Intervention by regulating communities through reducing alcohol availability, income quarantining, bans on pornography, removal of the permits systems and changes to the land tenure of communities. This example indicates the spatial aspect of 'government through community', as the measures were applied to 70-plus Aboriginal settlements in the Northern Territory as a whole without regard to each community's diversity and current processes for living well in place. This 'government through community' also takes on a new moral character and links individuals to their own self-responsibility while attributing certain affinity to the locality, family ties and cultural networks with an expectation that individuals are identified through close bonds (Miller & Rose, 2008).

'Each assertion of community refers itself to something that already exists and has a claim on us: our common fate as gay men, women of colour . . . residents in a village or a suburb,' argue Miller and Rose (2008: 92). This sentiment echoes Mae Shaw's (2008) point that policies locate problems with a 'community' and that these communities are 'contrived' and determined by policy-makers, often in relation to place-based location and an assumed affinity by individuals to a particular 'community' identity. From an anti-oppressive and empowerment perspective, the expectation that people identify with a 'contrived' community location or identity requires exploration to ascertain whether there is an oppressive impact in relation to these policy framings. In engaging with 'community' and community development projects, social workers need to carefully think through the mechanisms that are being used to position a 'community' in policy discourse, and also how the community is being required to position itself within the wider policy frameworks.

The 'whole-of-community' approach advocated here uses a critical ecological systems and governmentality approach to explore the recent 'growing interest in a wide range of governance engagements or partnerships between governments, citizens and communities' (Miller & Rose, 2008). There are a number of necessary conditions for such engagements, such as shared decision-making between the parties and mutual dependence between the partners—meaning that the power differences 'between those who actually engage in the processes should not be too large' (Bell & Hindmoor, 2009: 145). It is likely that a genuine approach to such state and community relations would require a substantial shift within the state, as well as a restructure that alters the state-centric nature of policy-making and resource distribution in relation to regional, rural and remote settings. The challenge may be that, in institutional terms, the relationship between government and 'community' is only rhetorically committed to community engagement and shared decision-making. This means that communities need to understand the limits of partnerships with governments while progressing how to live well in place beyond solely neo-liberal economic concerns.

Community development with a 'community as a whole' focus aims to engage in this complex task despite the fact that 'communities can be deeply fragmented and many local people support policies which would exacerbate rather than combat social exclusion' (Foley & Martin, 2000, cited in Bell & Hindmoor, 2009: 148). The common governmental expectation that communities 'will speak with one voice' is not realistic. Social workers from an anti-oppressive and empowerment perspective aim to work with community diversity in a way that facilitates processes which acknowledge these differences as well as the differential power relations between various groups. Clearly, social workers cannot approach a complex 'community as a whole' analysis and process by themselves or without engaging with a wide range of people, both locally and more widely. It is vitally important to develop and maintain relationships with various community members and groups, as well as with professionals from a variety of disciplines associated with specific settlements. In regional, rural and remote settings, interprofessional practice and interdependence between community members and experts is a necessary dimension for effective, enabling and empowering social work practice.

FOSTERING INTERDEPENDENCY

Several contributors to this book have referred to the integral role played by both formal and informal networks in rural regions when it comes to providing ongoing support to individuals, families and whole communities. Throughout, examples have been cited where synergies between civic, social, industry and agricultural interests have strengthened the collective fabric of communities, and where overlapping activities have blurred the boundaries between professional and lay endeavours, creating a milieu for responsive innovation and capacity-building (see the 'Don't wait, talk to a mate' program for addressing youth mental health in rural Victoria in Chapter 5, and the establishment of the West Wyalong group home for supported accommodation, with its coffee shop, gardening and recycling businesses employing people with disabilities in Chapter 7). Initiatives such as these provide alternative examples of practice interventions to those found in more urban settings, where organisational and governance infrastructure obligations tend to promote isolated silo-driven forms of service delivery, with more pronounced compliance and regulatory requirements. This is not to suggest that emergent local rural community initiatives lack accountability. Indeed, the nature of relationships between rural people who are friends and neighbours as well as business and professional contacts exacts a degree of personal and community accountability that sits beyond simply fulfilling compliance requirements.

Paradoxically, the scarcity of resources for health and social service delivery experienced on many levels in rural areas has created the impetus for developing innovative local solutions, such as those cited above. Through necessity, these initiatives are based on collaborative arrangements between community groups, service clubs and government organisations, professional and lay helpers, clients and workers. This way of working is only possible when the *interdependency* between people, disciplines, organisations, communities and environmental factors is acknowledged and utilised. In this tradition, a 'whole-of-community' response can be fashioned to address specific local issues.

For some, inducted into their discipline from an urban-centric educational base, the notion of promoting interdependency between professionals and with lay people is fraught. Acknowledgement of interdependency clearly challenges established traditional social relations and power differentials between the professions, and between the 'experts' and lay people. While the sociology of the professions traces the historical antecedents for the ways in which clear demarcations between professional groups have arisen (Macdonald, 1995), in an environment where resources, expertise and people power are restricted, there is limited utility to accommodate these sensibilities. Arguments about diluting the knowledge and skill base of individual professions are rendered redundant when a critical small-town industry closes its doors, signalling the potential slow death of a whole rural community.

Notwithstanding these pragmatic considerations, a growing body of evidence suggests that the state of interdependency, and of interdisciplinary knowledge and skill-sharing, is both necessary and more effective when it comes to addressing complex issues (Ellis, 2008). Such an approach offers the possibility of configuring new ways to address old problems, where exploring the liminal threshold areas—those spaces 'betwixt and between' the fringe of discipline borders—can yield potential ways forward (Turner, 1987, cited in Ellis, 2008: 9) in both service provision and new knowledge development. This paradigm offers particular opportunities for delivering rural social work, but requires practitioners to reconsider notions of teamwork, collaboration and networking within a critical ecological framework.

Fostering interdependent practice entails working alongside those professional and lay people in a community who store the local social, historical and familial knowledge; joining forces with workers from seemingly disparate or unrelated disciplines to develop innovative responses; and being mindful to preserve and restore the local ecology while also tapping into potential sources of constructive intervention offered up by the surrounding natural environment. While there has been little research on how the differing roles, status and expectations of lay and professional people working together impact upon team functioning, interdependency of this nature is prevalent in rural settings where community care and development responses are required to address local needs (McKee et al., 2010).

The niche for social work in this context is to help people to take action together to overcome the impacts of a crisis such as a business closure, a severe weather event or an outbreak of foot and mouth disease. The role of the practitioner is to facilitate inclusive collaborative action, mobilising aspects of the invisible economy, promoting resource-sharing, and stimulating policy advocacy. These actions are designed to protect and sustain the social, economic and ecological fabric of rural communities. Social work of this order is focused on fulfilling social-justice objectives. The process of valuing, protecting and sustaining local sources of ecological knowledge and practice is integral to promoting healthy forms of interdependent practice (Jones, 2010). In order to practise in this way, social workers need to be particularly informed about the nature, scope and impacts of changing community social and economic trends. Reading about, using and conducting social research to inform everyday practice is therefore critical in this context.

PRACTITIONER RESEARCH

Despite research commonly being cited and promoted as a critical social work task (Campbell & Fouche, 2009), there is plenty of evidence to suggest that practitioners are not necessarily confident about their own level of knowledge and skill in this area (Beddoe, 2010; Joubert, 2006). Ambivalence about engaging with research is a real barrier to using systematic inquiry for strengthening community needs analysis, service evaluation and policy advocacy initiatives. Nevertheless, development of practitioner research literacy is a priority for equipping social workers to advocate for change in an informed way, both now and in the future.

We read in Chapter 4 about how a housing shortage in one rural area was identified through research then addressed using the data in a submission for state funding to set up a local housing cooperative. In Chapter 8, we learned how research had been conducted in rural and remote Australian environments to identify some of the unique factors practitioners needed to be mindful of in their work with women subjected to violence. These are just two examples from many cited in this text where research has played an integral role in informing practice, while advocating for equitable resource distribution to rural communities.

While a great deal of literature in social work has been focused on promoting evidence-based practice (Yegidis & Weinbach, 2006; Grinnell & Unrau, 2008), we are not advocating this particular research paradigm at all. Instead, we believe rural practitioner research needs to be positioned within an anti-oppressive paradigm, with a focus on empowerment in practical ways, such as conducting community needs analysis and facilitating participatory action research. These processes serve to equip communities with the knowledge and skill base needed to promote macro policy change and service delivery development within their own regions. Such endeavours are not underscored by a desire to scientifically prove the worthiness of particular clinical interventions, but instead are designed to bring about transformative change for people and the communities in which they live. Examples of research efforts that reflect this approach are currently more prominent in community health, community psychology, environmental management and community practice than in social work (Santiago-Rivera et al., 1997; Minkler, 2005; Thomsen, 2008).

Traditionally, research activity has been given little priority in most social service agency settings, with demand for immediate responses to individual client issues taking precedence over developmental long-term change initiatives. A significant transformation in vision of what day-to-day social work can look like is required from practitioners, agency managers and service funders to reposition research as an integral practice activity. Demonstrating volumes of direct client contact has become critical in the current climate, where service contracts require agencies to meet funding provider targets. This model of measuring productivity and service delivery privileges a reactive band-aid approach to social work, and devalues developmental community-based work. Reconceptualising ideas about what activity comprises legitimate and effective service delivery requires policy-makers and those responsible for funding and management of services to see beyond the immediate feedback generated by the 'busyness' of direct practice. A change of focus of this order requires stakeholders to understand that the benefits of community-based research are not immediately obvious, and that this way of working necessitates a longer-term vision, a willingness to participate in power-sharing with the community, and a preparedness to withstand a short-term loss of direct client work capacity to achieve a long-term gain in community sustainability. In reality, research activity of this nature is a powerful medium for problem-solving and fostering change at the micro, meso *and* macro levels of intervention (Beddoe & Maidment, 2009).

This discussion leads us to consider how rural practitioners might equip themselves to engage in research—particularly in instances where they are geographically isolated and have not necessarily been encouraged to do so. We suggest four strategies that can be used to self-educate and facilitate research-mindedness in practice. The first involves using the internet, agency and local libraries to access and read articles, newsletters and online forums that discuss existing community-based research initiatives. Second, we suggest making email contact with practitioners (either within or outside social work) who identify as practitioner researchers. The purpose of this contact would be to inquire about the 'how to' for conducting research initiatives, ask about helpful resources and tips for engaging in community research, and to simply connect with others interested in this mode of practice. Third, practitioner research can be fostered through using face-to-face or online supervision and professional development opportunities to learn more about conducting research. Finally, becoming personally engaged with a local community development initiative that includes a research component is a grounded way to learn about this form of practice from real experience. Being curious and community-focused, proactive about information-seeking and knowledge development, and committed to policy advocacy are attributes that together encourage research-minded practice.

CONCLUSION

In this chapter, we have drawn together particular theoretical and practice principles for rural social work that have emerged out of the author contributions to this text. We are mindful that a publication of this nature cannot address every complexity that rural practitioners will inevitably face in their work. We are confident, however, that each chapter offers ways forward to creatively engage in rural community capacity-building in different fields of practice. We hope that this book will help to renew or awaken the desire among practitioners and students to discover more about rural living and working; raise questions about the legitimacy of traditional social work practice narratives; and encourage a deeper level of social work engagement with rural community concerns.

Rural social work is often credited with reminding social workers that social work itself is a contextual practice. Working in regional, rural and remote settings tends to highlight this contextual aspect of social work practice, and at times to stimulate reconceptualisations of social work practice itself. Social workers engage with theories, practice wisdom, analysis and understanding of the effects of their work when making sense of their day-to-day practice. This book offers insights into social work practice in a range of diverse community settings across Australia. Each chapter has highlighted ways to engage in social work practice contextually in order to promote 'living well in place'. The challenge of this century is for humanity to live well together in socially, ecologically and economically sustainable ways across the globe. Social work as a discipline has a significant role to play in helping to make this way of living and being in the world possible.

BIBLIOGRAPHY

ABC News (2010) WA to set up Mental Health Commission. Retrieved 29 March 2011 from <www.abc.net.au/news/stories/2010/02/04/2810532. htm>.

ACIL Tasman (2002) *Pathways to Profitability for Small and Medium Wineries.* Department of Agriculture, Fisheries and Forestry, Canberra. Retrieved 29 March 2011 from <www.daff.gov.au/agriculture-food/ hort-wine/wine-policy/domestic/pathways>.

Alber, G. (2011) *Gender, Cities and Climate Change.* Thematic report prepared for *Cities and Climate Change Global Report on Human Settlements* 2011. Retrieved 29 March 2011 from <www.unchs.org/ downloads/docs/GRHS2011/GRHS2011ThematicStudyGender.pdf>.

Allan, J. (2010) Determinants of mental health and well-being in rural communities: Do we understand enough to influence planning and policy? *Australian Journal of Rural Health*, 18, 3–4.

Allen, K. (2002) The social space(s) of rural women. *Rural Society*, 12(1), 27–45.

Alloway, N. & Dalley-Trim, L. (2009) High and dry in rural Australia: Obstacles to student aspirations and achievements. *Rural Society*, 19(1): 49–59.

Alston, M. (2004a) Social capital in rural Australia. *Rural Society*, 12(2), 93–104.

—— (2004b) Who is down on the farm? Social aspects of Australian agriculture in the 21st century. *Agriculture and Human Values*, 21(1), 37–46.

—— (2005a) Gender perspectives in Australian rural community life. In C. Cocklin & J. Dibden (eds), *Sustainability and Change in Rural Australia.* UNSW Press, Sydney, pp. 139–56.

—— (2005b) Social exclusion in rural Australia. In C. Cocklin & J. Dibden (eds), *Sustainability and Change in Rural Australia.* UNSW Press, Sydney, pp. 157–70.

—— (2009a) *Innovative Human Services Practice: Australia's changing landscapes.* Palgrave Macmillan, Sydney.

—— (2009b) Working with communities. In M. Connolly & L. Harms (eds), *Social Work: Contexts and practice*, 2nd edn. Oxford University Press, Melbourne, pp. 345–59.

—— (2010) Rural male suicide in Australia. *Social Science and Medicine*, in press.

Alston, M. & Kent, J. (2004) Dirt, drought, and drudge: Australian women's experience of drought. In E. Moore (ed.), *WOW, Wellbeing of Women*. Conference Proceedings, Community of Scholars, Gender, Women and Social Policy. Charles Sturt University, Wagga Wagga, NSW, pp. 71–81.

—— (2006) *Impact of Drought on Rural and Remote Education Access: A Report to DEST and Rural Education Fund of FRRR*. Centre for Rural Social Research, Charles Sturt University, Wagga Wagga, NSW.

—— (2009) Generation X-pendable: The social exclusion of rural and remote young people. *Journal of Sociology*, 45(1), 89–107.

Alston, M., Kent, J. & Kent, A. (2004) *Social Impacts of Drought: Report to NSW Agriculture*. Centre for Rural Social Research, Charles Sturt University, Wagga Wagga, NSW.

Alston, M., Whittenbury, K. & Dowling, J. (under review) Does climatic crisis in Australia's food bowl create a basis for change in agricultural gender relations? (Available from Department of Social Work, Monash University.)

Altman, J. (2009) No movement on the outstations. *Sydney Morning Herald*, 26 May. Retrieved 29 May 2011 from <www.culturalsurvival. org.au/ref_docs/No%20movement%20on%20the%20outstations.pdf>.

Ambrosino, R., Heffernan, J. & Shuttlesworth, G. (2008) *Social Work and Social Welfare: An introduction*, 6th edn. Thomson/Brooks Cole, Wadsworth, CA.

Anglicare (2004) *Non-completion of Year 12 Schooling: Incidence, reasons, impacts and programs*. Briefing paper, Anglicare Research and Planning Unit, Paramatta, NSW.

Atkinson, J. (2002) *Trauma Trails, Recreating Song Lines: The transgenerational effects of trauma in Indigenous Australia*. Spinifex, Melbourne.

Australian Association of Social Workers (AASW) (2010) *Code of Ethics*. Retrieved 28 May 2011 from <www.aasw.asn.au/publications/ethics-and-standards>.

Australian Bureau of Statistics (ABS) (2006) *A Picture of the Nation: The Statistician's Report on the 2006 Census*, cat. no. 2070.0. ABS, Canberra.

—— (2007a) *Australian Standard Geographical Classification*. Retrieved 20 May 2011 from <www.ausstats.abs.gov.au/Ausstats/subscriber.nsf/0

/00F66F76F2354DCECA2573630017AB54/$File/12160_jul%202007. pdf>.

—— (2007b) *Migration: Permanent additions to Australia's population.* Australian social trends, cat. no. 4102. Retrieved 20 May 2011 from <www.abs.gov.au/AUSSTATS/abs@.nsf/Latestproducts/928AF7A0CB6 F969FCA25732C00207852?opendocument>.

—— (2007c) *2006 Census Quickstats.* ABS, Canberra.

—— (2010a) *3218.0—Regional Population Growth, Australia, 2008–09.* Retrieved 18 October 2010 from <www.abs.gov.au/ausstats/abs@.nsf/ Products/3218.0~2008-09~Main+Features~Main+Features?OpenDocu ment#PARALINK3>.

—— (2010b) *Australian Demographic Statistics, Mar 2010,* cat. no. 3101.0. Retrieved 18 October 2010 from <www.abs.gov.au/ausstats/ abs@.nsf/mf/3101.0>.

Australian Council for Safety and Quality in Health Care (2005) *National Patient Safety Education Framework.* University of Sydney: The Centre for Innovation in Professional Health Education.

Australian Government (2007) *Australian Natural Resources Atlas.* Retrieved 18 October 2010 from <www.anra.gov.au>.

—— (2010a) *Closing the Gap: Prime Minister's Report 2010.* Commonwealth of Australia, Canberra. Retrieved 20 February 2011 from <www. fahcsia.gov.au/sa/indigenous/pubs/general/Pages/closing_the_gap_2010. aspx>.

—— (2010b) New and improved aircraft and mental health support service for Royal Flying Doctor. Press release, 5 February. Hon. Warren Snowden MP, Hon. Jenny Macklin MP, Hon. Jim Turnour MP.

—— (2010c) Continuing the fight against petrol sniffing. Press release, 10 November. Hon. Jenny Macklin and Hon. Warren Snowdon.

—— (2011) Mental health and wellbeing. Retrieved 18 October 2010 from <www.health.gov.au/internet/mentalhealth/publishing.nsf/Content/ home-1>.

Australian Health Ministers Advisory Council and National Rural Health Alliance (NRHA) (2002) *Healthy Horizons: Outlook 2003–07: A framework for improving the health of rural, regional and remote Australians, summary progress across Australia.* Australian Government Printing Service, Canberra.

Australian Human Rights Commission (AHRC) (2009) Sustaining Aboriginal homeland communities. In *Social Justice Report.* Retrieved 18 October 2010 from <www.humanrights.gov.au/social_justice/sj_ report/sjreport09/chap4.html>.

Australian Institute of Criminology (2010) *Australian Crime: Facts and Figures 2009*. Australian Institute of Criminology, Canberra. Retrieved 12 July 2010 from <www.aic.gov.au/statistics.aspx>.

Australian Institute of Health and Welfare (2007) *Older Australians at a Glance*, 4th edn. AIHW, Canberra. Retrieved 20 October 2010 from <www.aihw.gov.au/publications/age/oag04/oag04.pdf>.

—— (2009a) Disability and disability services. In *Australia's Welfare 2009*. Australia's welfare series no. 9. AIHW, Canberra, pp. 139–85.

—— (2009b) *Report Profile: Rural, Regional and Remote Health: Indicators of Health System Performance*. Retrieved 10 October 2010 from <www.aihw.gov.au/publications/phe/rrrh-ihsp/rrrh-ihsp-rp.pdf>.

—— (2010a) *Child Protection Australia 2008–09*. AIHW, Canberra.

—— (2010b) *A Profile of Social Housing in Australia*. AIHW, Canberra.

Bailie, R. & Wayte, K. (2006) Housing and health in Indigenous communities: Key issues for housing and health improvement in remote Aboriginal and Torres Strait Islander communities. *Australian Journal of Rural Health*, 14(5), 178–83.

Baltes, M. & Carstensen, L. (1996) The process of successful ageing. *Ageing and Society*, 16(4), 397–422.

Barbour, R.S., Stanley, N., Penhale, B. & Holden, S. (2002) Assessing risk: Professional perspectives on work involving mental health and child care services. *Journal of Interprofessional Care*, 16(4), 323–34.

Barclay, E., Foskey, R. & Reeve, I. (2007) *Farm Succession and Inheritance: Comparing Australian and international trends*. Rural Industries Research and Development Corporation, Canberra.

Barlow, M. (2007) *Blue Covenant: The global water crisis and the coming battle for the right to water*. Black Inc., Melbourne.

Barr, N. (2010) *The House on the Hill*. Halstead Press, Sydney and Land and Water Australia, Canberra.

Barr, N., Karunaratne, K. & Wilkinson, R. (2005) *Australian Farmers: Past, present and future*. Land and Water Australia, Canberra.

Barry, M.J. (1989) The role of the New South Wales Housing Commission in post-war reconstruction. *Australian Journal of Public Administration*, 48(3), 278.

Bauman, Z. (2000) *Community: Seeking safety in an insecure world*. Polity Press, Cambridge.

Bay, U. (2009) Framing critical social work practices with rural and remote communities. In J. Allen, L. Briskman & B. Pease (eds), *Critical Social Work: Theories and practices for a socially just world*, 2nd edn. Allen & Unwin, Sydney, pp. 268–80.

BBC News (2010) US 'Dr Death' jailed for seven years in Australia. Retrieved 1 July 2010 from <www.bbc.co.uk/news/10472261>.

Beddoe, E. & Maidment, J. (2009) *Mapping Knowledge for Social Work Practice: Critical intersections.* Cengage, Melbourne.

Beddoe, L. (2010) Continuing professional education in social work in New Zealand. Unpublished PhD thesis, Deakin University, Melbourne.

Beddoe, L. & Davys, A. (2008) Revitalizing supervision education through stories of confirmation and difference: The case for interprofessional learning. *Social Work Now,* 40, 34–41.

Beer, A., Tually, S., Rowley, S., Haslam McKenzie, F., Schlapp, J., Birdsall Jones, C. & Corunna, V. (2011) *The Drivers of Supply and Demand in Australia's Rural and Regional Centres.* AHURI Final Report No. 165. Australian Housing and Urban Research Institute, Melbourne.

Beeton, R., Buckley, K.I., Jones, G.J., Morgan, D., Reichelt, R.E. & Trewin, D. (2006) *State of the Environment.* Independent report to the Australian Government Minister for Environment and Heritage, Canberra.

Bell, R. (1973) *Mateship in Australia: Some implications for female–male relationships.* La Trobe University, Bundoora, Vic.

Bell, S. & Hindmoor, A. (2009) Governance through community engagement. In S. Bell & A. Hindmoor, *Rethinking Governance: The centrality of the state in modern society.* Cambridge University Press, Cambridge, pp. 137–61.

beyondblue (2011). Retrieved 20 March 2011 from <www.beyondblue.org.au>.

Bigby, C. (2008) Beset by obstacles: A review of Australian policy development to support ageing in place for people with intellectual disability. *Journal of Intellectual & Developmental Disability,* 33(1), 76–86.

Bigby, C. & Frawley, P. (2010) *Social Work Practice and Intellectual Disability.* Palgrave Macmillan, Basingstoke.

Black, A. (2005) Rural communities and sustainability. In C. Cocklin & J. Dibden (eds), *Sustainability and Change in Rural Australia.* UNSW Press, Sydney, pp. 20–37.

Blackstock, K. (2005) A critical look at community based tourism. *Community Development Journal,* 40(1), 39–49.

Blainey, G. (1966) *The Tyranny of Distance: How distance shaped Australia's history.* Sun Books, Melbourne.

Bland Shire Council (2011) *Bland Shire Council, West Wyalong.* Retrieved 10 February 2011 from <www.blandshire.nsw.gov.au>.

Bourke, L. (2001) One big happy family? Social problems in rural communities. In S. Lockie & L. Bourke (eds), *Rurality Bites: The social and environmental transformation of rural Australia.* Pluto Press, Sydney, pp. 89–102.

Bowles, W. (2005) Social work and people with disabilities. In M. Alston & J. McKinnon (eds), *Social Work Fields of Practice*, 2nd edn. Oxford University Press, Melbourne.

—— (2010) Reflections on rural identity from West Wyalong NSW. In N. Blacklow & T. Whitford (eds), *Where the Crows Fly Backward: Notions of rural identity*. Post Press, Brisbane.

Boxelaar, L., Paine, M. & Beilin, R. (2007) Sites of integration in a contested landscape. *Rural Society*, 17(3), 258–72.

Boyd, N.M. & Bright, D.S. (2007) Appreciate inquiry as a model of action research for community psychology. *Journal of Community Psychology*, 35(8), 1019–36.

Brems, C., Johnson, M.E., Warner, T.D. & Roberts, L. (2006) Barriers to healthcare as reported by rural and urban interprofessional providers. *Journal of Interprofessional Care*, 20(2), 105–18.

Briskman, L. (1999) Setting the scene: Unravelling rural practice. In L. Briskman & M. Lynn (eds), *Challenging Rural Practice: Human services in Australia*. Deakin University Press, Geelong, pp. 3–14.

—— (2007) *Social Work with Indigenous Communities*. Federation Press, Sydney.

Briskman, L. & Fiske, L. (2009) Working with refugees. In M. Connolly & L. Harms (eds), *Social Work: Contexts and Practice*, 2nd edn. Oxford University Press, Melbourne, pp. 135–48.

Briskman, L., Latham, S. & Goddard, C. (2008) *Human Rights Overboard: Seeking asylum in Australia*. Scribe, Melbourne.

Briskman, L., Pease, B. & Allan, J. (2009) Introducing critical theories for social work in a neo-liberal context. In J. Allan, L. Briskman & B. Pease (eds), *Critical Social Work: Theories and practices for a socially just world*, 2nd edn. Allen & Unwin, Sydney, pp. 1–14.

Brownlee, K., Graham, J.R., Doucette, E., Hotson, N. & Halverson, G. (2010) Have communication technologies influenced rural social work practice? *British Journal of Social Work*, 40(2), 622–37.

Bryant, L. & Pini, B. (2011) *Gender and Rurality*. Routledge, New York.

Bullock, S. (2010) Whose health? How population groups vary. In *Australia's Health 2010*. Australia's health series no. 12. AIHW, Canberra, Ch. 5.

Burnley, I. & Murphy, P. (2004) *Sea Change: Movement from Metropolitan to Arcadian Australia*. UNSW Press, Sydney.

Butera, K. (2008) 'Neo-mateship' in the 21st century: Changes in the performance of Australian masculinity. *Journal of Sociology*, 44(3), 265–81.

Butler, I., & Drakeford, M. (2005) *Scandal, Social Policy and Social Welfare*, 2nd edn. BASW Policy Press, Basingstoke.

Calma, T. (2008) The role of social workers as human rights workers with Indigenous people and communities. Social Work Orientation Week Seminar, Australian Catholic University. Retrieved 20 October 2010 from <www.hreoc.gov.au/about/media/speeches/social_justice/2008/20080212_socialwork.html>.

Campbell, L. & Fouche, C. (2009) Research in social work. In M. Connolly & L. Harms (eds), *Social Work: Contexts and practice*, 2nd edn. Oxford University Press, Melbourne, Ch. 28.

Carney, M. (2007) Tracking the intervention. *Four Corners*, ABC TV, 5 November.

—— (2008) The money pit. *Four Corners*, ABC TV.

Carrington, K. (1993) *Offending Girls: Sex, youth and justice*. Allen & Unwin, Sydney.

Carrington, K. & Marshall, N. (2008) Building social capital in regional Australia. *Rural Society*, 18(2), 117–30.

Cartwright, C. (2006) Investigating models of affordable housing for older people and people with disabilities in the Mid-North Coast Region of New South Wales. Southern Cross University, Lismore. Retrieved 18 April 2011 from <http://aslarc.scu.edu.au/Housing_ExecSumm.pdf>.

Cashmore, J. (2001) Child protection in the new millennium. *Social Policy Research Centre Newsletter*, 79, 1–5.

CBD, UNEP & IUCN (2007) *International Day for Biological Diversity: Biodiversity and climate change*. Retrieved 20 October 2010 from <www.biodiv.org>.

Chalmers, A.I. & Joseph, A.E. (2006) Rural change and the production of otherness: The elderly in New Zealand. In P. Cloke, T. Marsden & P. Mooney (eds), *Handbook of Rural Studies*. Sage, London, pp. 388–400.

Chambers, R. & Conway, G. (1992) *Sustainable Rural Livelihoods: Practical concepts for the 21st century*. Institute of Development Studies, Brighton.

Cheers, B., Darracott, R. & Lonne, B. (2007) *Social Care Practice in Rural Communities*. Federation Press, Sydney.

Cheers, B. & Taylor, J. (2005) Social work in rural and remote Australia. In M. Alston & J. McKinnon (eds), *Social Work Fields of Practice*, 2nd edn. Oxford University Press, Melbourne, pp. 237–48.

Chenoweth, L. & Stehlik, D. (2004) The implications of social capital for the inclusion of people with disabilities and families in community life. *International Journal on Inclusive Education*, 8(1), 59–72.

Clement, T. & Bigby, C. (2009) Breaking out of a distinct social space: Reflections on supporting community participation for people with severe and profound intellectual disability. *Journal of Applied Research in Intellectual Disabilities*, 22(3), 264–75.

Cocklin, C. & Alston, M. (2003) *Community Sustainability in Rural Australia: A question of capital in Australia*. Academy of Social Sciences, Canberra.

Cocklin, C. & Dibden, J. (eds) (2005) *Sustainability and Change in Rural Australia*. UNSW Press, Sydney.

Collins, J. (2010) Immigrants in rural and regional Australia: New arrivals and older legacies. Paper presented to NIRRA seminar. Retrieved 20 October 2010 from <www.nirra.anu.edu.au/event/nirra-seminar-12-march-immigrants-rural-regional-australia-new-arrivals-older-legacies>.

Collins, J., Winefield, H., Ward, L. & Turnbull, D. (2009) Understanding help seeking for mental health in rural South Australia: Thematic analytical study. *Australian Journal of Primary Health*, 15(2), 159–65.

Collis, M. (1999) Marital conflict and men's leisure: How women negotiate male power in a small mining community. *Journal of Sociology*, 35(1), 60–76.

Collits, P. & Gastin, B. (1997) Big town, small town: The centralisation of services and economic activity, the decline of small towns and policy responses in New South Wales. *Regional Policy and Practice*, 6(2), 9–21.

Commonwealth of Australia, Treasury (2002) *Intergenerational Report 2002–03*. Budget Paper no. 5.

——(2007) *Intergenerational Report*. Australian Government, April 2007.

——(2010) *Intergenerational Report, Australia to 2050: Future challenges*. Australian Government, January 2010.

Commonwealth Department of Health and Aged Care (2000) *LIFE: a framework for Prevention of Suicide and Self-Harm in Australia*. Mental Health and Special Programs Branch, Commonwealth Department of Health and Aged Care, Canberra.

Commonwealth Foundation (n.d.) *Putting Culture First*. Retrieved 22 April 2011 from <www.commonwealthfoundation.com/LinkClick.aspx?file ticket=HGliFtpmlS4%3d&tabid=313>.

Concerned Australians (2010) *This is What We Said: Australian Aboriginal people give their views on the Northern Territory Intervention*. Vega Press, Melbourne.

Cooke, B. & Kothari, U. (2001) *Participation: The new tyranny?* Zed Books, London.

Coombs, A. (2005) Mobilising rural Australia. *Griffith Review*, 3. Retrieved 20 October 2010 from <www.griffithreview.com/images/stories/edition_articles/ed3_pdfs/coombsed3.pdf>.

Corish, P. (2005) Equitable telecommunication service now and into the future. Paper presented to Australian Telecommunications Summit, Sydney, 22 November.

Council of Australian Governments (COAG) (2008) *National Partnership Agreement on Remote Service Delivery*. Retrieved 20 October 2010 from <www.coag.gov.au/intergov_agreements/federal_financial_relations/docs/national_partnership/national_partnership_on_remote_service_delivery_with_amended_schedule.rtf>.

—— (2009) *Fact Sheet—National Disability Agreement*. Retrieved 20 October 2010 from <www.coag.gov.au/coag_meeting_outcomes/2008-11-29/docs/20081129_national_disability_agreement_factsheet.pdf>.

—— (2010) *2010–2020 National Disability Strategy: An Initiative of the Council of Australian Governments*. Retrieved 20 October 2010 from <www.alp.org.au/agenda/more---policies/draft-national-disability-strategy>.

Crago, H. & Crago, M. (2002) But you can't get decent supervision in the country. In M. McMahon & W. Patton (eds), *Supervision in the Helping Professions: A practical approach*. Pearson Education, Sydney, pp. 79–90.

Crombie, A., Disler, P. & Threlkeld, G. (2009) Ageing in rural areas. In R. Nay & S. Garratt (eds), *Older People: Issues and innovations in care*. Elsevier, Sydney.

Crosby, E. (1998) Succession and inheritance on Australian family farms. Paper presented at the 6th Australian Institute of Family Studies Changing Families, Challenging Futures conference, Melbourne.

Culf, J. (2009) A big warm welcome: Building a stronger community through supporting new residents. *Rural Social Work and Community Practice*, 14(1), 42–6.

Cunneen, C. & Stubbs, J. (2007) *Migration, Political Economy and Violence Against Women: The post-immigration experiences of Filipino women in Australia*. Legal Studies Research Paper 07/25. University of Sydney Law School, Sydney.

Curtis, E. & Dixon, M. (2005) Family therapy and systemic practice with older people: Where are we now? *Journal of Family Therapy*, 27, 43–64.

Daley, M. & Avant, F. (2004) Rural social work: Reconceptualizing the framework for practice. In L. Scales & C. Streeter (eds), *Rural Social work: Building and sustaining community assets*. Thomson Brooks/Cole, Melbourne.

D'Amour, D., Ferrada-Videla, M., San Martin Rodriguez, L. & Beaulieu, M.D. (2005) The conceptual basis for interprofessional collaboration: Core concepts and theoretical frameworks. *Journal of Interprofessional Care*, 19(1), 116–31.

Davies, J. & Holcombe, S. (2009) Desert knowledge: Integrating knowledge and development in arid and semi-arid drylands. *GeoJournal*, 74, 363–75.

Davies, J., White J., Wright, A., Maru, Y. & LaFlamme, M. (2008) Applying the sustainable livelihoods approach in Australian desert Aboriginal development. *The Rangeland Journal*, 30(1), 55–65.

Davis, S. & Bartlett, H. (2008) Healthy ageing in rural Australia: Issues and challenges. *Australasian Journal on Ageing*, 27(2), 56–60.

Dean, J. & Stain, H. (2010) Mental health impact for adolescents living with prolonged drought. *Australian Journal of Rural Health*, 18, 32–7.

Department of Agriculture, Fisheries and Forestry (2010) *Domestic Fisheries.* Retrieved 18 October 2010 from <www.daff.gov.au/fisheries/domestic>.

Department of Health and Ageing (2010) National Alcohol Strategy 2006–2011. Retrieved 4 June 2010 from <www.alcohol.gov.au>.

Dibden, J. & Cocklin, C. (2005) Introduction. In C. Cocklin & J. Dibden (eds), *Sustainability and Change in Rural Australia*. UNSW Press, Sydney, pp. 1–18.

Disability Services Commission (2006) *Aboriginal People with Disabilities: Getting services right.* Government of Western Australia, Perth.

Dominelli, L. (2008) *Anti-racist Social Work*, 3rd edn. Palgrave Macmillan, New York.

Donzelot, J. (1979) *The Policing of Families*. Pantheon, New York.

Dunbar, J., Hickie, I., Wakerman, J. & Reddy, P. (2007) New money for mental health: Will it make things better for rural and remote Australia? *Medical Journal of Australia*, 186(11), 587–9.

Eacott, C. & Sonn, C. (2006) Exploring youth experiences of their communities: Place attachment and reasons for migration. *Rural Society*, 16(2), 199–214.

Eade, D. (1997) *Capacity Building: An approach to people-centred development.* Oxfam, Oxford.

Edwards, P. (2011) A landlord to call my own: More Australians are happy to remain tenants for life. *The Age*, Domain, 15 January, pp. 2–3.

Ellis, R. (2008) Problems may cut across the borders: Why we cannot do without interdisciplinarity. In B. Chandramohan, B. Fallows & S. Fallows (eds), *Interdisciplinary Learning and Teaching in Higher Education*. Routledge, Hoboken, NJ.

Erikson, E.H. (1982) *The Life Cycle Completed: A review*. W.W. Norton, New York.

European Commission (1996) *Cork Declaration—A Living Countryside.* Retrieved 20 October 2010 from <http://ec.europa.eu/agriculture/rur/cork_en.htm>.

Eversole, R. (2004) The industry gap in community development. *New Community Quarterly*, 2(1), 34–7.

Fabiansson, C. (2006) Being young in rural settings. *Rural Society*, 16(1), 47–60.

Falk, I. & Kilpatrick, S. (2000) What *is* social capital? A study of interaction in a rural community. *Sociologia Ruralis*, 1(40), 87–110.

Fawcett, B. & Waugh, F. (eds) (2008) *Addressing Violence, Abuse and Oppression: Debates and challenges*. Routledge, New York.

Finlay, S. & Dwyer, A. (2010) InterLink evaluation report. Unpublished report available from Chief Executive Officer, Kurrajong Waratah, PO Box 8576, Wagga Wagga, NSW 2650, Australia.

Food and Agricultural Organisation (FAO) (2007) *Gender and Climate Change: Existing research and knowledge gaps*. Gender and Population Division, FAO, Rome.

Fortescue Metals Group (2010) Fortescue Vocational Employment and Training Centre. Retrieved 4 June 2010 from <www.fmgl.com.au/irm/Community/index.html>.

Forth, G. (2001) Following the yellow brick road and the future of Australia's declining country towns. In M. Rogers & Y. Collins (eds), *The Future of Australia's Country Towns*. La Trobe University Press, Bendigo.

Foskey, R. (2005) *Older Farmers and Retirement*. Rural Industries Research and Development Corporation, Canberra.

Foucault, M. (1991) Governmentality. In G. Burchell, C. Gordon & P. Miller (eds), *The Foucault Effect: Studies in governmentality*. Harvester Wheatsheaf, London.

—— (2008) *The Birth of Biopolitics: Lectures at the College de France, 1978–1979*. A. Davidson (ed.). Palgrave Macmillan, New York.

Frost, W. (2006) From diggers to barristas: Tourist shopping villages in Victoria's goldfields. *Journal of Hospitality and Tourism Management*, 13(2), 136–43.

Garnaut, R. (2008) *The Garnaut Climate Change Review: Final report*. Cambridge University Press, Melbourne.

Garnett, A. & Lewis, P. (2007) Population and employment changes in regional Australia. *Economic Papers*, 26(1), 29–43.

Gething, L. (1997) Sources of double disadvantage for people with disabilities living in remote and rural areas of New South Wales, Australia. *Disability & Society*, 12(4), 513–31.

Gibson, C. (1994) Researching the 'divorce roster' with women in the coal communities of central Queensland. In M. Franklin, L. Short & E. Teather (eds), *Country Women at the Crossroads: Perspectives on the lives of rural Australian women in the 1990s.* University of New England Press, Armidale, NSW, pp. 63–75.

—— (2008) Reinventing rural places? The extent and impact of festivals as regeneration strategies. Retrieved 6 November 2010 from <www.uow.edu.au/science/eesc/eesstaff/UOW050077.html>.

Gibson, P. (2010) Working for the BasicsCard in the Northern Territory Emergency Response and associated policies on employment conditions in NT Aboriginal communities. In *Jumbunna Indigenous House of Learning.* University of Technology, Sydney, pp. 63–75.

Giddens, A. (2009) *The Politics of Climate Change.* Polity Press, Cambridge.

Gillard, J., Swan, W., Windsor, T. & Oakeshott, R. (2010) *The Australian Labor Party and the Independent Members (Mr Tony Windsor and Mr Rob Oakeshott) ('The Parties')—Agreement.* Parliament House, Canberra.

Gocher, K. (2010) Braidwood farmer looks to diversification. *ABC Rural,* ABC Radio. Retrieved 4 November 2010 from <www.abc.net.au/rural/content/2010/s3017816.htm>.

Gorman-Murray, A. (2009) What's the meaning of chillout? Rural/urban difference and the cultural significance of Australia's largest rural GLBTQ festival. *Rural Society,* 19(1), 71–86.

Graybeal, C. (2001) Strengths-based social work assessment: Transforming the dominant paradigm. *Families in Society: Journal of Contemporary Human Services,* 82(3), 233–43.

Green, R. (2003) Social work in rural areas: A personal and professional challenge. *Australian Social Work,* 56(3), 209–19.

Greene, R. (2008) *Social Work with the Aged and Their Families.* Transaction, New Brunswick, NJ.

Greene, R. & Kropf, N. (2009) *Human Behaviour Theory: A diversity framework,* 2nd rev. edn. Aldine Transaction, Piscataway, NJ.

Greenhill, J., King, D., Lane, A. & MacDougall, C. (2009) Understanding resilience in South Australian farm families. *Rural Society,* 19(4), 318–25.

Gregory, R., Green, R. & McLaren, S. (2007) The development of 'expertness': Rural practitioners and role boundaries. *Rural Social Work & Community Practice,* 12(2), 16–21.

Grewcock, M. (2009) *Border Crimes: Australia's war on illicit migrants.* Institute of Criminology, Sydney.

Grill, J. (2006) The case for and against the continued funding of remote Aboriginal communities: Report from the West. Paper presented to Bennelong Society Conference, Leaving Remote Communities. Retrieved

20 October 2010 from <www.bennelong.com.au/conferences/confer ence2006/Grill2006.php>.

Grinnell, R. & Unrau, Y. (2008) *Social Work Research and Evaluation: Foundation of evidence-based practice*. Oxford University Press, New York.

Hacking, I. (1991) The making and moulding of child abuse. *Critical Inquiry*, 17, 257–88.

Hall, G. & Scheltens, M. (2005) Beyond the drought: Towards a broader understanding of rural disadvantage. *Rural Society*, 15(2), 347–58.

Hall, P. (2005) Interprofessional teamwork: Professional cultures as barriers. *Journal of Interprofessional Care*, 19(2) (Supp. 1), 188–96.

Hall, P. & Weaver, L. (2001) Interdisciplinary education and teamwork: A long and winding road. *Medical Education*, 35, 867–75.

Hamilton, C. (2010) *Scorcher: The dirty politics of climate change*. Black Inc., Melbourne.

Handmer, J. & Dovers, S. (2009) A typology of resilience: Rethinking institutions for sustainable development. In L.F. Schipper & I. Burton (eds), *Adaptation to Climate Change*. Earthscan, London.

Harrison, J. & Lee, A. (2006) The role of e-health in the changing health care environment. *Nursing Economics*, 24(6), 283–9.

Harvey, D. (2009) Conceptualising the mental health of rural women: A social work and health promotion perspective. *Rural Society*, 19(4), 353–62.

Haxton, J.E. & Boelk, A.Z. (2010) Serving families on the frontline: Challenges and creative solutions in rural hospice social work. *Social Work in Health Care*, 49(6), 526–50.

Hayward, D. (1996) The reluctant landlords? The history of public housing in Australia. *Urban Policy and Research*, 14(1), 5–35.

Healy, K. (2005) *Social Work Theories in Context: Creating frameworks for practice*. Palgrave Macmillan, Basingstoke.

Healy, K. & Hampshire, A. (2002) Social capital: A useful concept for social work? *Australian Social Work*, 55(3), 227–38.

Healy, K. & Meagher, G. (2000) Cooperative and collective responses to market reform: Achieving recognition for professional human services. Paper presented to Managerialism, Contractualism and Professionalism in Human Services conference, Centre for Citizenship and Human Rights, Deakin University, Victoria, November.

Hegney, D., Gorman, D., McCullagh, B., Pearce, S., Rogers-Clark, C. & Weir, J. (2003) *Rural Men Getting Through Adversity: Stories of resilience*. Centre for Rural and Remote Health, University of Southern Queensland, Toowoomba, Qld.

Hicks, J., Basu, P.K. & Sappey, R. (2008) 55+ and working in an established rural regional Australian labour market. *Employment Relations Record*, 8(1), 1–16.

Higgs, J. & Jones, M. (eds) (2000) *Clinical Reasoning in the Health Professions*, 2nd edn. Butterworth Heinemann, Sydney.

Hocking, G. (2003) Oxfam Great Britain and sustainable livelihoods in the UK. *Community Development Journal*, 38(3), 235–42.

Hodgkin, S. (2010) Participating in the community: Are we all equal? *Australian Social Work*, in press.

Hogg, R. & Carrington, K. (2006) *Policing the Rural Crisis*. Federation Press, Sydney.

Horin, A. (2011) Rental squeeze hits hard as cheaper housing dries up. *Sydney Morning Herald*, Comments, 14 April, p. 52. Retrieved 17 April 2011 from <http://smh.domain.com.au/real-estate-news/rental-squeeze-hits-hard-as-cheaper-housing-dries-up-20110413-1de61.html>.

Hossain, D., Gorman, D., Eley, R. & Coutts, J. (2010) Value of mental health first aid training of advisory and extension agents in supporting farmers in rural Queensland. *Rural and Remote Health*, 10, 1593. Retrieved 20 October 2010 from <www.rrh.org.au/articles/subviewaust.asp?ArticleID=1593>.

Hughes, M. & Heycox, K. (2010) *Older People, Ageing and Social Work*. Allen & Unwin, Sydney.

Hugo, G. (2005) The state of rural populations. In C. Cocklin & J. Dibden (eds), *Sustainability and Change in Rural Australia*. UNSW Press, Sydney, pp. 56–79.

Human Rights and Equal Opportunity Commission (HREOC) (1997) *Bringing Them Home*. Report of the National Inquiry into the Separation of Aboriginal and Torres Strait Islander Children from Their Families. HREOC, Canberra. Retrieved 20 October 2010 from <www.human rights.gov.au/pdf/social_justice/bringing_them_home_report.pdf>.

—— (2008) *A Statistical Overview of Aboriginal and Torres Strait Islander Peoples in Australia*. Retrieved 20 October 2010 from <www.hreoc.gov. au/social_justice/statistics/index.html>.

Iacono, T., Davis, R., Humphreys, J. & Chandler, N. (2003) GP and support people's concerns and priorities for meeting the health care needs of individuals with developmental disabilities: A metropolitan and non-metropolitan comparison. *Journal of Intellectual & Developmental Disability*, 28(4), 353–68.

Ikuntji artists fine art from desert Australia. Retrieved 11 November 2010 from <www.ikuntji.com.au/aboutus/timeline/tabid/78/language/en-US/Default.aspx>.

Ingamells, A. (2007) Community development, community renewal: Tracing the workings of power. *Community Development Journal*, 42(2), 237–50.

Intergovernmental Panel on Climate Change (IPCC) (2007) *Fourth Assessment Report*. Retrieved 20 October 2010 from <www.ipcc.ch>.

Iverson, R. & Maguire, C. (2000) The relationship between job and life satisfaction: Evidence from a remote mining community. *Human Relations*, 53(6), 807–39.

Jackson, E. (2009) National Broadband Network: Rural and regional Australia. *Agribusiness Australia*. Retrieved 28 October 2010 from <www.agribusiness-australia.com.au/200912/national broadband>.

Jones, A., LaFleur, V. & Purvis, N. (2009) Double jeopardy: What the climate crisis means for the poor. In L. Brainard, A. Jones & N. Purvis (eds), *Climate Change and Global Poverty*. Brookings Institution Press, Washington, DC.

Jones, P. (2010) Responding to the ecological crisis: Transformative pathways for social work education. *Journal of Social Work Education*, 46(1), 67–84.

Joubert, L. (2006) Academic–practice partnerships in practice research: A cultural shift for health social workers. *Social Work in Health Care*, 43(2/3), 151–62.

Judd, F., Jackson, H., Fraser, C., Murray, G., Robins, G. & Komiti, A. (2006) Understanding suicide in Australian farmers. *Social Psychiatry & Psychiatric Epidemiology*, 41(1), 1–10.

Kelly, G. & Hosking, K. (2008) Non-permanent residents, place attachment, and 'sea change' communities, *Environment and Behavior*, 40(4), 575–94.

Kemshall, H. (2010) Risk rationalities in contemporary social work policy and practice. *British Journal of Social Work*, 40(4): 1247–62.

Kendig, H. (2000) Family change and family bonding in Australia. In W. Liu & H. Kendig (eds), *Who Should Care for the Elderly? An east–west divide*. Singapore University Press, Singapore.

Kenny, M. & Fiske, L. (2009) Social work practice with refugees and asylum seekers. In P. Swann & S. Rice (eds), *In the Shadow of the Law: The legal context of social work practice*, 3rd edn. Federation Press, Sydney, pp. 303–16.

Kenny, S. (2006) *Developing Community for the Future: Community development in Australia*, 3rd edn. Thomas Nelson, Melbourne.

Kesby, M. (2005) Retheorizing empowerment-through-participation as a performance in space: Beyond tyranny to transformation. *Signs: Journal of Women in Culture and Society*, 30(4), 2037–65.

Kilpatrick, S. & Abbott-Chapman, J. (2002) Rural young people's work/ study priorities and aspirations: The influence of family social capital. *The Australian Educational Researcher*, 29(1), 43–6.

Kingston, G., Tanner, B. & Gray, M. (2010) The functional impact of a traumatic hand injury on people who live in rural and remote locations. *Disability & Rehabilitation*, 32(4), 326–35.

Kirstein, K. & Bandranaike, S. (2004) *Rural Youth Drain: Attitudes, behaviours and perceptions*. Paper presented to the 12th Biennial Conference of the Australian Population Association, Canberra, 15–17 September.

Kurrajong Waratah (2011) *Kurrajong Waratah History*. Retrieved 20 October 2010 from <www.kurrajongwaratah.org.au/AboutUs/History. aspx>.

Langton, M. & Perkins, R. (eds) (2008) *First Australians: An illustrated history*. Melbourne University Publishing, Melbourne.

Lashlie, C. (2010) *The Power of Mothers*. HarperCollins, Auckland.

Légaré, F., Stacey, D., Pouliot, S., Gauvin, F.-P., Desroches, S., Kryworuchko, J. & Graham, I.D. (2011) Interprofessionalism and shared decision-making in primary care: A stepwise approach towards a new model. *Journal of Interprofessional Care*, 25(1), 18–25.

Locke, B., Garrison, R. & Winship, L. (1998) *Generalist Social Work Practice: Context, story and partnerships*. Brooks Cole, Belmont, CA.

Lockie, S. & Bourke, L. (2001) *Rurality Bites*. Pluto Press, Sydney.

Lonne, R. (2003) Social workers and human service practitioners. In M. Dollard, A. Winefield & H. Winefield (eds), *Occupational Stress in the Service Professions*. Taylor & Francis, London, pp. 281–310.

Lonne, R. & Cheers, B. (2001) Personal and professional adjustment of social workers to rural and remote practice: Implications for improved retention, issues affecting rural communities (II). In *Proceedings of the Rural Communities and Identities in the Global Millennium International Conference*. Nanaimo, British Columbia, Canada, pp. 48–53.

—— (2004) Retaining rural social workers: An Australian study. *Rural Society*, 14(2), 163–77.

Lovell, J. & Critchley, J. (2010) Women living in a remote Australian mining community: Exploring their psychological well-being. *Australian Journal of Rural Health*, 18, 125–30.

Macadam, R., Drinan, J., Inall, N. & McKenzie, B. (2004) *Growing the Capital of Rural Australia: The task of capacity building*. RIRDC Publication No 04/034. Rural Industries Research and Development Corporation, Canberra.

McCallum, D. (2009) Punishing welfare: Genealogies of child abuse. *Griffith Law Review*, 18(1), 114–28.

McColl, L. (2007) The influence of bush identity on attitudes to mental health in a Queensland community. *Rural Society*, 17(2), 107–24.

McDermott, R., O'Dea, K., Rowley, K., Knight, S. & Burgess, P. (1998) Beneficial impact of homelands movement on health outcomes in Central Australian Aborigines. *Australian and New Zealand Journal of Public Health*, 22(6), 653–8.

McDonald, C. (2006) *Challenging Social Work: The context of practice*. Palgrave Macmillan, Basingstoke.

Macdonald, K. (1995) *The Sociology of the Professions*. Sage, London.

McHugh, E. (2004) *Outback Heroes: Australia's greatest bush stories*. Penguin, Ringwood.

McKee, M., Kelley, M., Guirguis-Younger, M., MacLean, M. & Nadin, S. (2010) It takes a whole community: The contribution of rural hospice volunteers to whole person palliative care. *Journal of Palliative Care*, 26(2), 103–11.

MacKellar, D. (1971) 'My Country'. In *The Poems of Dorothea Mackellar*. Rigby, Sydney.

MacLeod, C.L. (2006) *Multiethnic Australia: Its history and future*. McFarland, Jefferson, NC.

McMichael, A.J. (2003) Global climate change and health: An old story writ large. In A.J. McMichael, D.H. Campbell-Lendrum, C.F. Corvalan, K.L. Eloi, A. Githeko, J.D. Scheraga & A. Woodward (eds), *Climate Change and Human Health: Risks and responses*. World Health Organization, Geneva.

Maidment, J. & Macfarlane, S. (2009) Debating the capacity of information and communication technology to promote inclusion. In A. Taket, B. Crisp, A. Nevill, G. Lamaro, M. Graham & S. Barter-Godfrey (eds), *Theorising Social Exclusion*. Routledge, London, pp. 95–104.

Markus, A., Jupp, J. & McDonald, P. (2009) *Australia's Immigration Revolution*. Allen & Unwin, Sydney.

Marsh, P. (2006) Promoting children's welfare by inter-professional practice and learning in social work and primary care. *Social Work Education*, 25(2), 148–60.

Martin, J. (2006) Social work with refugees and asylum seekers. In W.H. Chui & J. Wilson (eds), *Social Work and Human Services Best Practice*. Federation Press, Sydney.

Mason, R. (2007) Building women's social citizenship: A five-point framework to conceptualise the work of women-specific services in rural Australia. *Women's Studies International Forum*, 30(4), 299–312.

—— (2009) A future for rural social work in Victoria: Developing a framework for working in uncertainty. *Rural Social Work & Community Practice*, 14(1), 48–56.

Mason, R., O'Mahony, B. & Deery, M. (2008) The food and wine trail: Domesticating a hybrid. In Council for Australasian University Tourism and Hospitality Education, *Where the Bloody Hell Are We?* Griffith University, Gold Coast, pp. 1–13.

Mearns, R. & Norton, A. (eds) (2010) *Social Dimensions of Climate Change: Equity and vulnerability in a warming world.* World Bank, Washington. Retrieved 20 October 2010 from <http://web.worldbank.org/WBSITE/EXTERNAL/TOPICS/EXTSOCIALDEVELOPMENT/0,,contentMDK:22408501~pagePK:210058~piPK:210062~theSitePK:244363,00.html>.

Miller, P. & Rose, N. (2008) *Governing the Present.* Polity Press, Cambridge.

Minkler, M. (2005) Community based research partnerships: Challenges and opportunities. *Journal of Urban Health*, 82(2), 1–2.

Molnar, J.J. (2010) Climate change and social response: Livelihoods, communities and the environment. *Rural Sociology*, 75(1), 1–16.

Moran, M. & Elvin, R. (2009) Coping with complexity: Adaptive governance in desert Australia. *GeoJournal*, 74, 415–28.

Moreton-Robinson, A. (2000) *Talkin' Up to the White Woman: Indigenous women and feminism.* University of Queensland Press, Brisbane.

Morgan, P. (2007) Policy considerations for moderating welfare dependency amongst rural youth. *Rural Society*, 18(1), 51–63.

Mullaly, B. (2002) *Challenging Oppression: A critical social work approach.* Oxford University Press, Toronto.

Mullen, C., Maguire, S., Plummer, N., Jones, D. & Creighton, C. (2010) Talking climate change with the bush. In I. Jubb, P. Holper & W. Cai (eds), *Managing Climate Change: Papers from the GREENHOUSE 2009 Conference.* CSIRO Publishing, Melbourne, pp. 249–57.

Munford, R., Nash, M. & O'Donoghue, K. (2005) *Social Work Theories in Action.* Jessica Kingsley, London.

Murray, G., Judd, F., Jackson, H., Fraser, C., Komiti, A., Hodgins, G. & Robins, G. (2004) Rurality and mental health: The role of accessibility. *Australian & New Zealand Journal of Psychiatry*, 38(8), 629–34.

Nancarrow, H., Lockie, S. & Sharma, S. (2009) *Intimate Partner Abuse of Women in a Central Queensland Mining Region.* Report No. 378. Criminology Research Council, Canberra.

National Council to Reduce Violence Against Women and Their Children (NCRVAWTC) (2009) *Time for Action 2009–2021.* NCRVAWTC, Canberra.

National People with Disabilities and Carers Council (2009) *Shut Out: The Experience of People with Disabilities: National Disability Strategy Consultation Report.* Commonwealth of Australia, Canberra.

National Rural Health Alliance (NRHA) (2011) *Health Reform—2007 to the present*. Retrieved 17 February 2011 from <http://nrha.ruralhealth. org.au>.

National Shelter (2011) *Housing Australia Factsheet: A quick guide to housing facts and figures*. Shelter, Sydney. Retrieved 1 April 2011 from <www.shelter.org.au/archive/fly-factsheet-australia.pdf>.

Naughtin, G. & Schofield, V. (2009) Working with older people. In M. Connolly & L. Harms (eds), *Social Work: Contexts and Practice*. Oxford University Press, Melbourne.

Neumayer, E. & Pluemper, T. (2007) The gendered nature of natural disasters: The impact of catastrophic events on the gender gap in life expectancy 1981–2002. Retrieved 20 October 2010 from <www2. lse.ac.uk/geographyAndEnvironment/whosWho/profiles/neumayer/pdf/ Disastersarticle.pdf>.

New South Wales Department of Human Services: Ageing, Disability and Home Care (2008) *Guidelines for the Support Coordination Program: Facilitating Support and Social Networks for Older Parent Carers*. NSW Government, Sydney.

—— (2009) *Annual Report 2009/10*. NSW Government, Sydney.

New South Wales Farmers Mental Health Network (NSWFMHN) (2006) *NSW Farmers Blueprint for Maintaining the Mental Health and Well-being of the People on NSW Farms*. Retrieved 20 October 2010 from <www.aghealth.org.au/blueprint/index.html>.

New South Wales Ombudsman (2010) *Improving Service Delivery to Aboriginal People with a Disability: A Review of the Implementation of ADHC's Aboriginal Policy Framework and Aboriginal Consultation Strategy*. NSW Ombudsman, Sydney.

New South Wales Parliament Standing Committee on Social Issues (2003) *Report on Community Housing*. NSW Parliament, Sydney.

Nimmo, J. & Zubrycki, T. (2008) *The Intervention, Katherine, NT* (video recording). Screen Australia and New South Wales Film and Television Office/Australian Broadcasting Corporation/Jotz Productions.

Nipperess, S. & Briskman, L. (2009) Promoting a human rights perspective on critical social work. In *Critical Social Work: Theories and practices for a socially just world*, 2nd edn. Allen & Unwin, Sydney, pp. 58–69.

Northcott Disability Services (2011) *About Us*. Retrieved 20 October 2010 from <www.northcott.com.au/about_us.php>.

Northern Territory Government (2010) *Growing Them Strong, Together: Promoting the safety and wellbeing of the Northern Territory's children*. Summary Report of the Board of Inquiry into the Child Protection System in the Northern Territory 2010, M. Bamblett, H. Bath & R. Roseby, Northern Territory Government, Darwin.

Nossal, K. and Gooday, P. (2009) Raising productivity growth in Australian agriculture, ABARE Research Report, *Issues Insights* 09.7, Canberra.

Oandasan, I. & Reeves, S. (2005) Key elements for interprofessional education. Part I: The learner, the educator and the learning context. *Journal of Interprofessional Care*, 19, 21–38.

Onyx, J., Edwards, M. & Bullen, P. (2007) The intersection of social capital and power: An application to rural communities. *Rural Society*, 17(3), 215–30.

Onyx, J., Wood, C., Bullen, P. & Osburn, L. (2005) Social capital: A rural youth perspective. *Youth Studies Australia*, 24(4), 21–7.

O'Toole, K., Schoo, A. & Hernan, A. (2010) Why did they leave and what can they tell us? Allied health professionals leaving rural settings. *Australian Health Review*, 34(1), 66–72.

Our Generation: Land Culture Freedom (2011) Retrieved 4 July 2011 from <www.ourgeneration.org.au/resources>.

Panelli, R. (2006) Rural society. In P. Cloke, T. Marsden, & P. Mooney (eds), *Handbook of Rural Studies*. Sage, London, pp. 63–90.

Parsons, L. & Stanley, M. (2008) The lived experience of occupational adaptation following acquired brain injury for people living in a rural area. *Australian Occupational Therapy Journal*, 55(4), 231–8.

Parton, N. (1991) *Governing the Family: Child care, child protection and the state*. Macmillan, Basingstoke.

Passant, J. (2009) The Socceroos, strikes and 'un-Australian' activities. *Sydney Morning Herald*, 21 October.

Payne, M. (2005) Systems and ecological perspectives. In *Modern Social Work Theory*, 3rd edn. Palgrave Macmillan, Basingstoke.

Peet, R. & Watts, M. (eds) (2004) *Liberation Ecologies, Environment, Development, Social Movements*. Routledge, London.

Perera, S. (2007) *Our Patch: Enacting Australian sovereignty post-2001*. Curtin University of Technology, Perth.

Petkova, V., Lockie, S., Rolfe, J. & Ivanova, G. (2009) Mining developments and social impacts on communities: Bowen Basin case studies. *Rural Society*, 19(3), 211–28.

Pierce, D., Liaw, S.T., Dobell, J. & Anderson, R. (2010) Australian Football club leaders as mental health advocates: An investigation of the Coach the Coach project. *International Journal of Mental Health Systems*, 4, 10.

Piper, M. and Associates (2009) *Regional Humanitarian Settlement Pilot: Ballarat*. Report of an evaluation undertaken for DIAC, Commonwealth of Australia, Canberra.

Productivity Commission (2005) Trends in Australian Agriculture, research paper, Canberra. <www.pc.gov.au/_data/assets/pdf_file/0018/8361/agri culture.pdf>.

Proudley, M.A. (2008) Fire, families and decisions. Unpublished Master of Applied Science thesis, RMIT University, Melbourne.

Pugh, R. & Cheers, B. (2010) Rural Social Work: An international perspective. Policy Press, Bristol.

Putnam, R. (2000) Making Democracy Work: Civic traditions in modern Italy. Princeton University Press, Princeton, NJ.

Quinlan, E. & Robertson, S. (2010) Mutual understanding in multidisciplinary primary health care teams. Journal of Interprofessional Care, 34(5), 565–78.

Rawsthorne, M. (2008) Violence against women in rural settings. In B. Fawcett & F. Waugh (eds), Addressing Violence, Abuse and Oppression: Debates and challenges. Routledge, London, pp. 93–105.

Reeve, C. (1994) Migrant women in the north west mining towns of Western Australia. In M. Franklin, L. Short & E. Teather (eds), Country Women at the Crossroads: Perspectives on the lives of rural Australian women in the 1990s. University of New England Press, Armidale, NSW, pp. 76–83.

Refugee Council of Australia (RCOA) (2010) Economic, Civic and Social Contributions of Refugees and Humanitarian Entrants: A literature review. Prepared for the Department of Immigration and Citizenship, February.

Regional Development Victoria (2010) Ready for Tomorrow: A blueprint for regional and rural Victoria. Retrieved 21 December 2010 from <www.rdv.vic.gov.au/ready-for-tomorrow/blueprint>.

Robertson, K. (2011) Door open to wider clientele: A modified co-operative housing model could be the answer for people who thought the dream was over. The Age, Domain, 12 March, pp. 10–11.

Roces, N. (2003) Sisterhood is local: Filipino women in Mount Isa. In N. Piper & N. Roces (eds), Wife or Worker? Asian women and migration. Rowman and Littlefield, Lanham, MD, pp. 73–100.

Rogers, M. & Ryan, R. (2001) The triple bottom line for sustainable community development. Local Environment Journal, 6(3), 279–89.

Rose, D. & Farrow, J. (2009) Perspectives on drug use. In M. Connolly & L. Harms (eds), Social Work: Contexts and practice, 2nd edn. Oxford University Press, Melbourne, pp. 248–61.

Rothery, M. (2008) Critical ecological systems theory. In N. Coady & P. Lehmann (eds), Theoretical Perspectives for Direct Social Work Practice: A generalist-eclectic approach, 2nd edn. Springer, New York, pp. 89–118.

Rudd, K., Tanner, L. & Conroy, S. (2010) Joint media release. Agreement between NBN and Telstra on the rollout of the National Broadband Network. Retrieved 28 October 2010 from <www.minister.dbcde.gov.au/media/media_releases/2010/060>.

Rule, A. & Silvester, J. (2010) It's un-Australian: 'Wychie' struggling to keep its GP, is up in arms over plans to sell off its pharmacy. *Sydney Morning Herald*, 16 October.

Rural Doctors Association of Australia (RDAA) (2010) *Measuring Remoteness: Classification systems and their application across rural and remote Australia*. Retrieved 28 October 2008 from <www.rdaa.com.au/Uploads/Documents/Measuring%20remoteness%20-%20Classification%20systems%20and%20their%20application%20across%20rural%20and%20remote%20Australia_20101012030513.pdf>.

Rural Industries Research and Development Corporation (RIRDC) & Australian Centre for Agricultural Health and Safety (ACAHS) (2008) *The Mental Health of People on Australian Farms: The facts*. RIRDC & ACAHS, Canberra.

Saleebey, D. (ed.) (2002) *The Strengths Perspective in Social Work Practice*, 3rd edn. Allyn and Bacon, Boston.

Salt, R. (2009) Trimming the list for a tree change. *The Australian*. Retrieved 20 October 2010 from <www.theaustralian.com.au/business/property/trimming-the-list-for-a-tree-change/story-e6frg9gx-1111118465128>.

Sanders, W. & Holcombe, S. (2007) Sustainable governance for small desert settlement: Learning from the multi-settlement regionalism of Anmatjere Community Government Council. *The Rangeland Journal*, 30(1), 137–47.

Santiago-Rivera, A., Morse, G., Hunt, A. & Lickers, H. (1997) A new paradigm in community research: Lessons from a Native American community. *Journal of Community Psychology*, 26, 163–74.

Sartore, G.-M., Kelly, B., Stain, H., Albrecht, G. & Higginbotham, N. (2008) Control, uncertainty, and expectations for the future: A qualitative study of the impact of drought on a rural Australian community. *Rural and Remote Health*, 8, 950. Retrieved 20 October 2010 from <www.rrh.org.au/articles/subviewaust.asp?ArticleID=950>.

Satour, J. (2009) Transport needs: Legitimising voices of Alice Springs Aboriginal town camp residents, unpublished Honours thesis, Deakin University, Waurn Ponds, Vic.

Schwarten, E. (2010) Couple jailed for sex slavery in Cairns Supreme Court. *Courier-Mail*, 18 February. Retrieved 4 June 2010 from <www.couriermail.com.au/news/queensland/couple-jailed-for-sex-slavery-in-cairns-supreme-court/story-e6freoof-1225831887543>.

Scoones, I. (2009) Livelihoods perspectives and rural development. *Journal of Peasant Studies,* 36(1), n.p.

Scott, B. (2011) Coffs housing getting expensive. *Coffs Coast Advocate,* 1 February. Retrieved 17 April 2011 from <www.coffscoastadvocate. com.au/story/2011/02/01/coffs-harbour-housings-become-too-expen sive>.

Scott, D., Arney, F. & Vimpani, G. (2010) Think child, think family, think community. In F. Arney & D. Scott (eds), *Working with Vulnerable Families: A partnership approach.* Cambridge University Press, Melbourne, pp. 7–28.

Senate Select Committee on Housing Affordability (2008) *A Good House is Hard to Find: Housing affordability in Australia.* Commonwealth of Australia, Canberra.

Setterland, D., Wilson, J. & Tilse, C. (2006) Older people. In W. Chui & J. Wilson (eds), *Social Work and Human Services Best Practice.* Federation Press, Sydney, pp. 150–71.

Sharma, S. & Rees, S. (2007) Consideration of the determinants of women's mental health in remote Australian mining towns. *Australian Journal of Rural Health,* 15, 1–7.

Shaw, A. (2011) Home is where the matrix is: In a remarkable achievement, a social group for lesbians can now offer affordable housing to older women. *MCV,* 537, 7.

Shaw, M. (2008) Community development and the politics of community. *Community Development Journal,* 43(1), 24–36.

Sherwood, P. (2000) Diversity: The fibre of a vibrant rural town in Western Australia—Nannup. *Social Alternatives,* 19(4), 38–43.

Short, D. (2010) Australia: A continuing genocide. *Journal of Genocide Research,* 12(1), 45–68.

Shortall, S. (2004) Social or economic goals, civic inclusion or exclusion? An analysis of rural development theory and practice. *Sociologia Ruralis,* 44(1), 109–23.

Silverstein, M. & Bengston, V. (1997) Intergenerational solidarity and the structure of adult child–parent relationships in American families. *Journal of Sociology,* 103, 429–60.

Simmons, G. (2003) From the bush to the mall. *Australian Education Online,* 33. Retrieved 21 October 2010 from <http://search.informit. com.au/documentSummary;dn=820917907660155;res>.

Simpson, M.C. (2009) An integrated approach to assess the impacts of tourism on community development and sustainable livelihoods. *Community Development Journal,* 44(2), 186–208.

Sivamalai, S. & Nsubuga-Kyobe, A. (2009) Towards developing personal attributes in 'new' migrants: A case study of capacity building for rural Australia. In *Proceedings from the International Unity Diversity Conference: People, the Workforce & the Future of Australia*, Townsville.

Smith, J. (2010) Paralympian, Motivational Speaker. Retrieved 2 February 2011 from <http://jessicasmith.com.au>.

Smith, R. (2008) *Social Work and Power*. Palgrave Macmillan, Basingstoke.

Smith, R. & Anderson, L. (2008) Interprofessional learning: Aspiration or achievement? *Social Work Education: The International Journal*, 27(7), 759–76.

Smith, T. (2008) The letter, the spirit, and the future: Rudd's apology to Australia's Indigenous people. *Australian Review of Public Affairs*. Retrieved 20 October 2010 from <www.australianreview.net/digest/2008/03/smith.html>.

Sparrow, P. & Thomson, F. (2004) *Affordable Housing for Older People: A Literature Review*. Aged and Community Services, Melbourne. Retrieved 20 October 2010 from <www.agedcare.org.au/POLICIES-&-POSITION/Position-and-discussion-papers/affordable_housing_a_literature_review_final.pdf>.

Spencer, M., Gunter, K. & Palmisano, G. (2010) Community health workers and their value to social work. *Social Work*, 55(2), 169–80.

Squires, C. & Gurran, N. (2005) Planning for affordable housing in coastal sea change communities. *Proceedings of Building for Diversity, National Housing Conference*, pp. 381–403. Retrieved 20 October 2010 from <www.nhc.edu.au/downloads/2005/Refereed/20Squires.pdf>.

Stanley, N. & Manthorpe, J. (eds) (2004) *The Age of the Inquiry: Learning and blaming in health and social care*. Routledge, London.

Stayner, R. (2005) The changing economics of rural communities. In C. Cocklin & J. Dibdin (eds), *Sustainability and Change in Rural Australia*. UNSW Press, Sydney, pp. 121–38.

Stehlik, D. (2009) Intergenerational transitions in rural Western Australia: An issue for sustainability. In F. Merlan (ed.), *Tracking Rural Change: Community, policy and technology in Australia, New Zealand and Europe*. ANU e-Press, Canberra, pp. 135–50.

Stratton, J. (2009) Preserving white hegemony. Skilled migration, 'Asians' and middle-class assimilation. *Borderlands e-journal*, 8(3). Retrieved 13 May 2010 from <www.borderlands.net.au/vol8no3_2009/stratton_hegemony.htm>.

Sydney Morning Herald (2006) Migrants need to learn mateship: PM. 12 December.

Tedmanson, D. & Wadiwel, D. (2010) Neoptolemus: the governmentality of new race/pleasure wars? *Culture and Organization*, 16(1), 7–22.

Thompson, A. & Gullifer, J. (2006) Subjective realities of older male farmers: Self-perceptions of ageing and work. *Rural Society*, 16, 80–97.

Thompson, N. (2006) *Anti-discriminatory Practice*, 4th edn. Palgrave Macmillan, Basingstoke.

Thomsen, D. (2008) Community based research: Facilitating sustainability learning. *Australasian Journal of Environmental Management*, 15(4), 222–30.

Thorpe, D. (1994) *Evaluating Child Protection*. Open University Press, Buckingham.

Tilse, C., Rosenman, L., Peut, J., Ryan, J., Wilson, J. & Setterlund, D. (2006) Managing older people's assets: Does rurality make a difference? *Rural Society*, 16(2), 169–85.

Tonna, A., Kelly, B., Crockett, J., Grieg, J., Buss, R., Roberts, R. & Wright, M. (2009) Improving the mental health of drought-affected communities: An Australian model. *Rural Society*, 19(4), 296–305.

Tonts, M. (2005) Government policy and rural sustainability. In C. Cocklin & J. Dibden (eds), *Sustainability and Change in Rural Australia*. UNSW Press, Sydney, pp. 194–211.

Tribe, D. (2005) What's happening to agriculture?: The benefits of technological transitions. *Institute of Public Affairs Review*, 57(4), 20–3.

United Nations (2008) Convention on the Rights of Persons with Disabilities. Retrieved 20 September 2010 from <www.un.org/disabilities/default.asp?navid=13&pid=150>.

—— (2010) *Backgrounder: Disability Treaty Closes a Gap in Protecting Human Rights*. Retrieved 28 January 2010 from <www.un.org/disabilities/default.asp?id=476>.

Victorian Department of Community Services & Fogarty, J. (1991) *Confidential Report of the Ministerial Panel of Inquiry into the Death of Daniel Valerio*. Victorian Government, Melbourne.

Victorian Department of Human Services (VDHS) (2003) *Protecting Children: The Child Protection Outcomes Project—Final Report of the Victorian Department of Human Services Melbourne, Community Care Division*. Retrieved 20 October 2010 from <www.dhs.vic.gov.au/pdpd/pdfs/finalreport.pdf>.

Walsh, J. (2010) *Theories for Direct Social Work Practice*, 2nd edn. Wadsworth Cengage, Belmont, CA.

Warburton, J. & McLaughlin, D. (2005) Lots of little kindnesses: Valuing the role of older Australians as informal volunteers in the community. *Ageing & Society*, 25, 715–30.

Warr, D. (2005) Social networks in a 'discredited' neighbourhood. *Journal of Sociology*, 41(3), 285–308.

Webster, B. (2008) 'They'd go out of their way to cover up for you': Men and mateship in the Rockhampton Railway Workshops. *History Australia*, 4(2), 43.1–43.15.

Weeks, W., Hoatson, L. & Dixon, J. (eds) (2003) *Community Practices in Australia*. Pearson, Sydney.

Wendt, S. (2009) *Domestic Violence in Rural Australia*, Federation Press, Sydney.

Wenger, E., McDermott, R. & Synder, W. (2002) *Cultivating Communities of Practice*. Harvard University Business School Press, Cambridge, MA.

West Pilbara Communities for Children (2010) Retrieved 4 June 2010 from <www.wpc4c.org.au/default.aspx?WebpageID=1>.

Whiteside, M. (2004) The challenge of interdisciplinary collaboration in addressing the social determinants. *Australian Social Work*, 57(4), 381–93.

Wild, R. & Anderson, P. (2007) *Ampe Akelyernemane Meke Mekarle: Little Children Are Sacred. Report of the Northern Territory Board of Inquiry into the Protection of Aboriginal Children from Sexual Abuse.* Northern Territory Government, Darwin.

Wilkinson, J. (2005) *Affordable Housing in NSW: Past to present.* Briefing Paper No. 14/05. NSW Parliamentary Library, Sydney, pp. 1–54.

Williams, C. (1981) *Open Cut: The working class in an Australian mining town.* Allen & Unwin, Sydney.

Williams, J. & Lakhani, N. (2010) E-learning for interprofessional education: A challenging option. *Journal of Interprofessional Care*, 24(2), 201–3.

Winterton, R. & Warburton, J. (2010) Does place matter? Reviewing the experience of disadvantage for rural older populations. *Rural Society*, under review.

Women's Services Network (WESNET) (2000) *Domestic Violence in Regional Australia: A literature review.* Partnerships Against Domestic Violence, Canberra.

Woods, M. (2005) *Rural Geography.* Sage, London.

Woolcock, M. & Narayan, D. (2000) Social capital: Implications for development theory, research and policy. *World Bank Research Observer*, 15(2), 225–49.

World Commission on Environment and Development (WCED) (1987) *Our Common Future* (The Brundtland Report), Oxford University Press, Oxford.

World Health Organization (WHO) (2010) *Framework for Action on Interprofessional Education and Collaborative Practice.* WHO, Geneva.

Yegidis, B. & Weinbach, R. (2006) *Research Methods for Social Workers*, 5th edn. Pearson, New York.

Young, M. & Guenther, J. (2008) The shape of Aboriginal learning and work opportunities in desert regions. *The Rangeland Journal*, 30(1), 177–86.

Youngt, A.E., Strasser, R. & Murphy, G.C. (2004) Agricultural workers' return to work following spinal cord injury: A comparison with other industry workers. *Disability & Rehabilitation*, 26(17), 1013–22.

Zapf, M. (1993) Remote practice and culture shock: Social workers moving to isolated northern regions. *Social Work*, 38(6), 694–704.

—— (2009) *Social Work and the Environment: Understanding people and place*. Canadian Scholars' Press, Toronto.

Zhao, Y., Condon, J.R., Guthridge, S. & Jiqiong, Y. (2010) Living longer with a greater health burden: Changes in the burden of disease and injury in the Northern Territory Indigenous population between 1994–1998 and 1999–2003. *Australian & New Zealand Journal of Public Health*, 34, S93–S98.

INDEX